The Capital Grille 28

Captain D's Seafood Kitchen 29

Carino's Italian Restaurant..30

Carl's Jr 31

Carrabbas 32

Charley's Grilled Subs..33

Charlie Brown's Steakhouse 34

Cheeseburger in Paradise 35

Cheesecake Factory 37

Chick-Fil-A 38

Chili's..39

Chipotle 41

Claim Jumper..42

The Coffee Bean and Tea Leaf 43

Cold Stone Creamery 44

Cosi..46

Cracker Barrel Old Country Store..47

Culver's..49

Dairy Queen 50

Dave and Buster's 51

Denny's 53

Disclaimer: We do not guarantee, nor do these restaurants guarantee that any menu item will be 100% gluten-free. These restaurants & Business Graphics Group assume no liability for your use of this information. See full disclaimer on page 7.

Dunkin Donuts (beverage info)	55
Eat 'n Park	56
El Pollo Loco	58
Firehouse Subs	59
First Watch	60
Five Guys Burgers and Fries	62
Fleming's Prime Steakhouse & Wine Bar	63
Friendly's	65
Golden Corral	67
Hardee's	69
In-N-Out Burger	70
Islands Restaurant	71
Jamba Juice	72
Jersey Mike's Subs	73
Johnny Rockets	74
Kentucky Fried Chicken	76
Krystal	77
Legal Sea Foods	78
Logan's Roadhouse	80
LongHorn Steak House	82
Long John Silver's	84

Disclaimer: We do not guarantee, nor do these restaurants guarantee that any menu item will be 100% gluten-free. These restaurants & Business Graphics Group assume no liability for your use of this information. See full disclaimer on page 7.

Macaroni Grill 85

Max & Erma's 87

McAlister's Deli 88

McDonalds 89

Melting Pot 91

Mitchell's Fish Market 92

Moe's Southwest Grill 94

Morton's The Steakhouse 95

Ninety-Nine Restaurants 96

Noodles & Company 97

The Old Spaghetti Factory 98

Olive Garden 99

On The Border Mexican Grill 100

Outback Steakhouse 102

Panera Bread 104

Pei Wei Asian Diner 106

P.F. Chang's China Bistro 107

Pizza Fusion: 108

Potbelly Sandwich Shop 109

Qdoba Mexican Grill 110

Quiznos: 111

Disclaimer: We do not guarantee, nor do these restaurants guarantee that any menu item will be 100% gluten-free. These restaurants & Business Graphics Group assume no liability for your use of this information. See full disclaimer on page 7.

- Red Lobster 112
- Red Robin 114
- Rubio's Fresh Mexican Grill 116
- Ruby Tuesday 117
- Salad Creations 119
- Shane's Rib Shack 120
- Sizzler 121
- Smokey Bones Bar and Fire Grill 123
- Sonic 124
- Starbucks 126
- Subway 127
- Taco Bell 128
- Ted's Montana Grill 129
- Tony Roma's 131
- Uno's Chicago Grill 132
- Wendy's 133
- Wingstop 135

Disclaimer: We do not guarantee, nor do these restaurants guarantee that any menu item will be 100% gluten-free. These restaurants & Business Graphics Group assume no liability for your use of this information. See full disclaimer on page 7.

Why is this book important?

The Gluten-Free Market

- 1 in 100 Americans have Celiac Disease, and require a 100% gluten-free diet
- 15 to 25 percent of consumers report looking for gluten-free products
- An estimated 6-10 million people are choosing a gluten-free lifestyle for reasons other than Celiac Disease such as autism spectrum disorders and gluten sensitivities
- Gluten intolerance is growing and many people find that following a gluten-free diet gives them better health in general
- The gluten-free community is a strong and well-connected group that regularly share dining out experiences with each other
- Gluten-free folks will travel a long way for a safe and delicious meal become loyal customers to restaurants with clear gluten-free menus
- Restaurants who offer gluten-free selections and menus have reported a 14% increase in business

---

Disclaimer: We do not guarantee, nor do these restaurants guarantee that any menu item will be 100% gluten-free. These restaurants & Business Graphics Group assume no liability for your use of this information. See full disclaimer on page 7.

Introduction and Disclaimer

Gluten Free Road Food: Your guide to eating wheat and gluten-free on the go.

This guide includes gluten-free menu items from the nation's top chain restaurants.

We have compiled this list of publicly available information and email responses to help you navigate life without gluten and wheat and discover that more and more establishments understand the importance of providing allergen information to their customers. Many of these restaurants now offer a gluten free menu, so please check with your server to see if one is available – and always inform the staff of your dietary needs and allergies.

Disclaimer: Whether you were diagnosed with a wheat or gluten intolerance or Celiac Disease ten minutes ago, or ten years ago, one of the first things you learn is that YOU are ultimately responsible for ensuring your own dietary safety. This guide is intended to serve as a resource for gluten-free menu options based on publically available information. We cannot and do not guarantee that ANY restaurant food item is 100% gluten free due to changing ingredients, suppliers, recipes, staff and the likelihood for cross contact or cross contamination. If food is cooked with, in, or even next to other gluten-containing items, your food may not be gluten-free. Cautious diners should verify this information, and contact restaurant managers or guest relations before dining as information changes frequently. Use this list as a guide only. You must take 100% responsibility and eat at your own risk.   Please note that we do not guarantee, nor do these restaurants guarantee that any food you order from this list will be 100% gluten-free, but we have used this guide successfully to eat without gluten while on the road and hope you can too!

Gluten Free Road Food, its publisher and the listed restaurants do not assume any liability for your use of this information. Guests with any special food sensitivities or dietary needs should <u>not</u> rely solely on this information as the basis for deciding whether to consume a particular menu item, and are individually responsible for ensuring that any such menu item meets their individual dietary requirements. Every reasonable effort has been made to make this book as accurate as possible given changing information. However, we acknowledge the possibility of mistakes that may be typographical or related to content. Use this book as a guide only and always discuss your diet choices with your physician.

Disclaimer: We do not guarantee, nor do these restaurants guarantee that any menu item will be 100% gluten-free. These restaurants & Business Graphics Group assume no liability for your use of this information. See full disclaimer on page 7.

Abuelo's

The following information about gluten-free menu items has been obtained either from the restaurant's website or through direct contact with guest services via email or phone.

Gluten Intolerance

A few of our menu items can be adjusted to accommodate a gluten free diet, but none fully meet the criteria. We can suggest the following menu items as gluten free. We also invite you to speak with your server or one of our managers while dining in our restaurant. There may be some other menu items you may enjoy.

Spring Mix Salad with no dressing
Steamed broccoli
Tortilla Soup with no grated cheese or tortilla chips
Salmon San Carlos with no sauce
Steak, Chicken, Shrimp, Pork or Vegetable Fajitas served without tortillas

Abuelo's General Nutritional Statement

Our menu consists of many new and exciting items that change quite often throughout the year – and all of our menu items are made fresh daily from premium ingredients. Due to the fresh nature of our recipes, specifications for the preparation of our items can vary based on the variances of the fresh product and, therefore, actual nutritional content may vary. As such, we are unable to provide detailed information or specific nutritional analysis for all the items on our menu.

We can, however, provide you with some suggestions for guests who may be interested in specific menu options including lower calorie, lower fat, lower carb or vegetarian menu options. As we are a full-service kitchen, we are happy to make substitutions or modify menu offerings to help meet your specific diet preferences. When dining with us, just ask a manager or your server to assist you.

Disclaimer: We do not guarantee, nor do these restaurants guarantee that any menu item will be 100% gluten-free. These restaurants & Business Graphics Group assume no liability for your use of this information. See full disclaimer on page 7.

Applebee's

As America's Favorite Neighbor, the health and safety of our guests are top priorities at Applebee's. Our commitment to you is to provide the most current allergen information available from our food suppliers. The menu items listed on this page are not prepared with wheat or made with ingredients that contain wheat when prepared according to the standard recipe. Please be aware that during normal kitchen operations involving shared cooking and preparation areas, including common fryer oil, the possibility exists for food items to come in contact with other food products. **Due to these circumstances, we are unable to guarantee that any menu item can be completely free of allergens.**

List of Wheat-Free Menu Items (gluten is not listed on their allergen chart):

Appetizers:
Buffalo Chicken Wings, no Sweet & Spicy Sauce
Chips & Salsa
Potato Skins
Queso Blanco Dip

Salads without Dressing:
Asian Crunch Salad
Blackened Chicken Salad
Grilled Shrimp 'N Spinach
Santa Fe Chicken Salad
Paradise Chicken Salad

Salad Dressings:
Ranch
Creamy Bleu Cheese
Fat-Free Italian
Garlic Caesar Dressing
Honey Balsamic
Honey French
Honey Mustard
Hot Bacon Honey Mustard
Mexi Ranch
Oriental Vinaigrette
Thousand Island
Non-Fat Balsamic Vinaigrette
Russian Dressing

Desserts
Hot Fudge Sundae

Seafood:
Not Including Sides
Grilled Shrimp & Island Rice
Cajun Lime Tilapia

Chicken:
Not Including Sides
Grilled Dijon Chicken & Portobello
Fiesta Lime Chicken
Margherita Chicken
Smothered Grilled Chicken
Garlic Herb Chicken

Sides:
Baked Potato - regular & loaded
French Fries
Cole Slaw
Fruit Side
Garlic Mashed Potatoes -regular & loaded,
Seasonal Vegetables
Almond Rice Pilaf
Weight Watchers® Rice
Island Rice
Mexi Rice
Celery, Applesauce
Weight Watchers® Herb Potatoes
Add Grilled Shrimp

Steaks:
Not Including Sides
Bourbon Street Steak
New York Strip
Ribeye

Steak Toppers:
Grilled Onions
Shrimp 'N Parmesan

Sauces:
Pico de Gallo
Honey Barbecue
Southern Barbecue
Guacamole
Tartar Sauce
Seafood Sauce
Garlic Herb Butter
Parmesan Topping
Chipotle Mayo
Marinara
Wing Sauce
Salsa
Bruschetta
Balsamic Glaze
Creamy Avocado Dressing
Balsamic Mayo
Black Bean Corn Salsa
Dijon Sauce
Signature Slider Sauce
A.1.® Sauce
Mayonnaise
Sour Cream

Disclaimer: We do not guarantee, nor do these restaurants guarantee that any menu item will be 100% gluten-free. These restaurants & Business Graphics Group assume no liability for your use of this information. See full disclaimer on page 7.

Applebee's Continued:

Every effort is made to keep this information current. However, it is possible that ingredient changes and substitutions may occur due to the differences in regional suppliers, product changes, preparation techniques, and/or the season. Certain menu items may vary from restaurant to restaurant and may not be available at all locations. We recommend that our guests with food allergies or special dietary needs consult with a restaurant manager prior to placing an order to review the posted information for accuracy and availability at that particular location. Limited time offers, test products, and regional items are not included in the posted information. Since this information expires on a QUARTERLY basis, please be sure you are referencing the most current version. Because of the individualized nature of allergies and food sensitivities, Applebee's cannot make recommendations that are suitable for your dietary needs. Please consult your physician

---

Disclaimer: We do not guarantee, nor do these restaurants guarantee that any menu item will be 100% gluten-free. These restaurants & Business Graphics Group assume no liability for your use of this information. See full disclaimer on page 7.

Arby's

Ingredient information is based on standard product formulations. Variations may occur due to differences in suppliers, ingredient substitutions, recipe revisions, product assembly at the restaurant level, and/or the season of the year. Certain menu items may not be available at all locations. Temporary products are not included. This information is effective as of November 2009. Arby's Restaurant Group, Inc., its franchisees and employees do not assume responsibility for a particular allergy or sensitivity to any food provided in our restaurants. We encourage anyone with food allergies, sensitivities, or special dietary needs to check our website at www.arbys.com on a regular basis to obtain the most comprehensive and up-to-date information. If you have specific questions about our menu, call or write: Arby's Restaurant Group, Inc., 1155 Perimeter Center West, Atlanta, GA 30338, 1-800-487-2729.

Arby's® U.S. Menu Items without Gluten (*No Wheat, Barley, Oats, or Rye*)

Meats:
Corned Beef
Genoa Salami
Pecan Chicken Salad-Roast+
Pepper Bacon
Pepperoni
Roast Beef
Roast Chicken+
Roast Ham
Roast Turkey

Beverages:
1% Low Fat Chocolate Milk
2% Reduced Fat Milk
CapriSun®
Coffee
Diet Blackberry Iced FruiTea
Diet Dr Pepper®*
Diet Mountain Dew®*
Diet Peach Iced FruiTea
Diet Pepsi®
Dr Pepper®
Mandarin Peach Iced FruiTea
Mountain Dew®
Mug® Root Beer*
Orange Juice*
Passion Fruit Iced FruiTea
Pepsi®

Salads:
Chopped Turkey Club
Chopped Farmhouse Chicken-Roast
Chopped Italian Salad
Chopped Side Salad*

Dressings:
Balsamic Vinaigrette
Buttermilk Ranch
Dijon Honey Mustard

Breakfast:
Breakfast Bacon
Breakfast Syrup
Egg, Scrambled Patty
Egg, Scrambled Mix
Sausage Patty

Desserts:
Chocolate Swirl Shake
Jamocha Swirl Shake
Vanilla Shake

Dipping Sauces:
Arby's Sauce®
Bronco Berry Sauce®*
Buffalo Dipping Sauce
Honey Dijon Mustard Sauce
Horsey Sauce®
Marinara Sauce

Sides:
Applesauce

Condiments:
Banana Peppers
Bleu Cheese Spread
Chargrill Seasoning
Cheddar Cheese Sauce+
Cheddar, Sharp Natural Slice
Cheddar, Shredded
Cheddar, Processed Slice
Chicken Club Sauce
Dijon Honey Mustard
Sandwich Sauce
Dill Pickles
Garlic Buttered Onions
Gyro Sauce
Gyro Seasoning
Ketchup
Mayonnaise
Parmesan Peppercorn Ranch Sauce
Pepper & Onion Mix
Red Ranch Sauce
Red Wine Vinaigrette Sauce
Sauerkraut
Smoky Q Sauce*
Spicy Brown Honey

Disclaimer: We do not guarantee, nor do these restaurants guarantee that any menu item will be 100% gluten-free. These restaurants & Business Graphics Group assume no liability for your use of this information. See full disclaimer on page 7.

Arby's Continued:

Sierra Mist®
SoBe® Energy*
Sweet Tea
Tropicana® Fruit Punch*
Tropicana® Light Lemonade*

Ranch Dipping Sauce
Spicy Three Pepper® Sauce+*
Tangy Barbeque Sauce
Tangy Southwest Sauce®*

Mustard Sauce
Swiss Cheese, Big Eye Natural
Swiss Cheese, Slice Processed
Tartar Sauce*
Thousand Island Spread
Yellow Mustard

Potato Cakes & Homestyle Fries* may be cooked in the same oil as Crispy Chicken Fillets, Crispy Chicken Tenders*, Curly Fries, Fish Fillets, Jalapeno Bites®, Loaded Potato Bites®, Mozzarella Sticks, Onion Petals, & Popcorn Chicken which contain a wheat allergen.

Pepsi, Diet Pepsi, Mountain Dew, Sierra Mist, Mug, SoBe, and Diet Mountain Dew are registered trademarks of PepsiCo Inc. Dr Pepper and Diet Dr Pepper are registered trademarks of Dr Pepper/Seven Up, Inc. CapriSun is a trademark of the Deutsche SiSi-Werke GmbH & Co. Betriebs KG. Tropicana is a registered trademark of Tropicana Products, Inc.
*Certain menu items may vary from store to store and may not be available at all locations.
+Contains maltodextrin from a corn source.

This list may not be published or distributed in any manner without prior written consent of Arby's Restaurant Group, Inc. TM & © 2009 Arby's IP Holder Trust

---

Disclaimer: We do not guarantee, nor do these restaurants guarantee that any menu item will be 100% gluten-free. These restaurants & Business Graphics Group assume no liability for your use of this information. See full disclaimer on page 7.

Austin Grill

The following information about gluten-free menu items has been obtained either from the restaurant's website or through direct contact with guest services via email or phone.

Gluten-Free Menu: Our kitchens are not exclusively gluten-free. We make every effort to avoid cross contamination, but that cannot be guaranteed.

Appetizers:
Austin Wings
Longhorn Nachos: Steak, Chicken or Combo
Quesadillas: Chicken or Spinach & Portobello
Guacamole

Salads and Soups:
Grilled Steak Wedge Salad
Southwest Caesar Salad - Grilled Chicken, Steak, Shrimp or Salmon for an additional price
Austin Chopped Salad - Add Grilled Chicken for an additional price
Shrimp and Avocado Salad
Bevo Salad - Add Grilled Chicken, Steak, Shrimp or Salmon for an additional price
Grilled Salmon Salad served with an Austin Grill potato
Mexican Corn Soup
Tortilla Soup

Combo Platters:
Austin Taco Combo -. *Must substitute corn tortilla*
Classic Combo - *Must substitute corn tortilla*

Mesquite Grill:
Austin Pesto Chicken
Rib Eye Steak
Slow Smoked BBQ Ribs
Grilled Red Snapper
Pan Seared Salmon
Pork Chop

Texas Favorites:
Tacos al Carbon - *Must substitute corn tortilla*
Carnitas Tacos - *Must substitute corn tortilla*
Red Snapper Tacos - *Must substitute corn tortilla*
Grilled Chicken Tacos - *Must substitute corn tortilla*
Fajitas - Must substitute corn tortillas. Choose from: Marinated Skirt Steak, Grilled Chicken Breast, Grilled Shrimp, Carnitas, Grilled Vegetables or a Combination
Pollo Guisado - *Must substitute corn tortilla*
Enchiladas Cheese or Spinach, Chicken or Beef Barbacoa, Shrimp or Austin Special.

Dessert:
Giffords Ice Cream: Available in Mexican vanilla, chocolate, toasted coconut and cinnamon.

Locations

919 Ellsworth Drive
Silver Spring, MD 20910
240-247-8969

750 E Street
Washington, DC 20004
202-393-3776

2400 Boston Street
Baltimore, MD 21224
410-534-0606

36 Maryland Avenue
Rockville, MD 20850
301-838-4281

8430 Old Keene Mill Rd.
Springfield, VA 22152
703-644-3111

2002 Annapolis Mall
Annapolis, MD 21404
410-571-6688

801 King Street
Alexandria, VA 22314
703-684-8969

Disclaimer: We do not guarantee, nor do these restaurants guarantee that any menu item will be 100% gluten-free. These restaurants & Business Graphics Group assume no liability for your use of this information. See full disclaimer on page 7.

Backyard Burgers

The following information about gluten-free menu items has been obtained either from the restaurant's website or through direct contact with guest services via email or phone.

Burgers:
Back Yard American Cheeseburger – *no bun*
Back Yard American Cheeseburger, Jr. – *no bun*
Back Yard Bleu Cheeseburger – *no bun*
Back Yard Bleu Cheeseburger Jr. – *no bun*
Back Yard Burger – *no bun*
Back Yard Burger, Jr. – *no bun*
Back Yard Cheddar Cheeseburger – *no bun*
Back Yard Cheddar Cheeseburger, Jr. – *no bun*
Back Yard Pepper Jack Cheeseburger – *no bun*
Back Yard Pepper Jack Cheeseburger, Jr. – *no bun*
Back Yard Swiss Cheeseburger – *no bun*

Back Yard Swiss Cheeseburger, Jr. – *no bun*
Bacon Cheddar Burger – *no bun*
Black Jack Burger – *no bun*
Mushroom Swiss Burger – *no bun*

Salads:
Blackened Chicken Salad – *no croutons*
Garden Fresh Salad – *no croutons*
Grilled Chicken Salad – *no croutons*

Sides:
Chili
Side Salad

Condiments:
Dressing, Honey Mustard
Dressing, Balsamic Vinaigrette
Dressing, Bleu Cheese (contains msg)
Dressing, Ranch (contains msg)
Dressing, Ranch, Lite (contains msg)
Margarine Cup
Mayonnaise, Light, Packet
Mayonnaise, Real, Packet

Chicken Sandwiches:
Blackened Chicken – *no bun*
Grilled Chicken – *no bun*

Specialty Items:
Back Yard Big Dog – *no bun*

Back-Pak Dog – *no bun*

Chili Cheese Big Dog – *no bun*

Desserts and Shakes:
Shake, Chocolate
Shake, Strawberry
Shake, Vanilla

Drinks:
Lemonade
Tea, Sweetened
Tea
sugar
Tea, Unsweetened
Dr. Pepper
Dr. Pepper, Diet
Mt Dew
Mug Root Beer
Pepsi
Pepsi, Diet
Sierra Mist
Sobe Lean Cranberry Grapefruit
Tropicana Fruit Punch

Disclaimer: We do not guarantee, nor do these restaurants guarantee that any menu item will be 100% gluten-free. These restaurants & Business Graphics Group assume no liability for your use of this information. See full disclaimer on page 7.

Bertucci's Italian Restaurant

This menu and the information on it are provided by Bertucci's Italian Restaurant, in cooperation with the Gluten Intolerance Group® (GIG®), as a service to our guests. Bertucci's assumes no responsibility for its use and any resulting liability or consequential damages are denied. Our management teams and service staff are not trained on the intricacies of Celiac Disease or Gluten intolerance and cannot be expected to provide recommendations or other advice on the issue. All questions and requests for recommendations should be directed to Bertucci's corporate office. Patrons are encouraged to consider the information provided, to their own satisfaction, in light of their individual needs and requirements. Prices and items may vary by location and are subject to change. GF 11/09

Appetizers:
Shrimp Scampi Appetizer - *Order without grilled crostini*
Mussels Caruso - *Order without grilled crostini*
Antipasto Misto

Salads:
Salad Vivaldi con Pollo & Bello
Insalata
Tomato & Mozzarella Caprese Salad
Caesar Salad- *Order without garlic croutons*
Grilled Chicken Chopped Salad
Venetian Spinach Salad with Grilled Chicken
Salad Giardino with Grilled Chicken

Entrées:
Grilled Steak & Chicken Combo
Filet Mignon with Chianti Sauce
Balsamic Chicken
Pollo Sanremo with half Insalata
Grilled Salmon Fillet*
Salmon Florentine
Eggplant Parma with String Beans

Soup:
Sausage Soup

Side Dishes:
Spinach & Artichokes
Broccoli Romana
Red Skin Mashed Potatoes
Roasted Tuscan Vegetables
Fresh Asparagus
String Beans

Desserts:
Bomba and Chocolate Budino

Disclaimer: We do not guarantee, nor do these restaurants guarantee that any menu item will be 100% gluten-free. These restaurants & Business Graphics Group assume no liability for your use of this information. See full disclaimer on page 7.

Biaggi's Ristorante Italiano

The following information about gluten-free menu items has been obtained either from the restaurant's website or through direct contact with guest services via email or phone.

Gluten Free Menu

Appetizers:
Carpaccio (*Please specify no flatbread grissini when ordering.*)
Mussels in Tomato-Garlic Broth (*Please specify no grilled baguette crouton when ordering.*)
Tomato Mozzarella Caprese

Salads:
House Salad
Caesar Salad (*Please specify no croutons when ordering.*)
Spinach Salad (Please specify no Gorgonzola cheese when ordering.)
Messina Salad
Chopped Chicken Salad (*Please specify no Gorgonzola cheese when ordering.*)
Venetian Chicken Salad (*Please specify no Gorgonzola cheese when ordering.*)
Seared Salmon Salad

Gluten Free Pasta:
Capellini Di Mare
Rigatoni Alla Toscana
Farfalle Alfredo
Linguini and Clams
Spaghetti Marinara

Entrees:
Grilled Chicken Parmesean
Grilled Chicken Pietro
Salmon & Shrimp Milanese
Seared Sea Bass
Chicken Piemontese
Grilled Pork Chops (*Specify no Parmesan-Gorgonzola butter when ordering.*)
N.Y. Strip
Filet Mignon

Gluten-Free Sauces:

Alfredo	Marsala	Scallion Cream
Bolognese	Pesto	Sun-Dried Tomato Cream
Espresso Sauce	Roasted Red Pepper Cream	Tomato Sauce
Italian Salsa	Rum Caramel	Mac & Cheese Sauce

Pizza: Made with our Gluten-Free dough
Chicken Piccante, Sausage Pizza, Pepperoni Pizza, Margherita Pizza, Mediterranean Pizza

---

Disclaimer: We do not guarantee, nor do these restaurants guarantee that any menu item will be 100% gluten-free. These restaurants & Business Graphics Group assume no liability for your use of this information. See full disclaimer on page 7.

BJ's Restaurant & Brewhouse

BJ's menu is diverse and contains a wide variety of foods, many of which contain one of the eight major allergens. While we have carefully reviewed our recipes to inform our guest of foods that contain a food allergen as part of a recipe, we cannot guarantee that cross-contact with other foods will not occur during production. Please inform your server if you, or any of the guests in your dining party, have any food allergies. The following information is provided for our guests who have food and allergen sensitivities or an intolerance to gluten. This information was obtained from published sources and suppliers of each of the items. Please inform your server if you, or any of the guests in your dining part, have any food allergies.

Great Beginnings:
Crisp Potato Skins Platter
Spinach & Artichoke Dip
Chips & Salsa
Chicken Wings

Garden Fresh Specialty Salads:
Santa Fe Salad
Italian Market Salad
Field of Greens
Garden Medley Salad
House Wedge Salad
House Salad (*no croutons*)
House Caesar Salad (*no croutons*)
BBQ Chicken Chopped Salad (*no onion strings*)

Soup:
Tuscan Tomato Bisque (*no croutons*)

Giant Stuffed Potatoes:
Garden Vegetable Potato (*no Alfredo sauce*)
Blackened Chicken Potato (*no Alfredo sauce*)
Grilled Chicken Potato (*no Alfredo sauce*)
The "Classic" Baked Potato

Specialty Entrees:
Flame Broiled New York Strip
Fresh Atlantic Salmon (*no rice pilaf*)
Roasted Chicken
Balsamic Glazed Chicken (*no onion strings*)

Weekend Brunch:
BJ's California Scramble (*no toast*)
Scrambled Egg Breakfast (*no toast*)

Breakfast Sides:
Country Sausage Links, Grilled Ham & Applewood Smoked Bacon

Disclaimer: We do not guarantee, nor do these restaurants guarantee that any menu item will be 100% gluten-free. These restaurants & Business Graphics Group assume no liability for your use of this information. See full disclaimer on page 7.

Bonefish Grill

The following information about gluten-free menu items has been obtained either from the restaurant's website or through direct contact with guest services via email or phone.

Starters & Sharing:
Saucy Shrimp
Mussels Josephine

Greens:
Bonefish Caesar
Bonefish House
Chilled Asparagus
Grilled Salmon and Asparagus Salad
Florida Cobb Salad

Vegetables and Sides
Garlic Whipped Potatoes
Herbed Jasmine Rice
Steamed Vegetable Medley
French Green Beans
Steamed Broccoli

Grilled Fish:
Gulf Grouper
Snake River Rainbow Trout
Chilean Sea Bass
Atlantic Salmon
Ahi Tuna
Sea Scallops & Shrimp
Longfin Tilapia
Cold Water Lobster Tails

*Seasonal Vegetable Garnish served with all entrees is Gluten Free (except Zucchini and Tomatoes)

Signature Sauces:
Mango Salsa
Chimichurri *(GF if ordered without the Aji Panca rub)*
Lemon Butter

Grilled Specialties:
Lily's Chicken
Sirloin Steak
Filet Mignon

Desserts:
Macadamia Nut Flourless
Crème Brulée with berries and whipped cream

Martinis and Cocktails:
Black Cherry Guava Mojito
Lemongrass Martini
Pomegranate Martini
Ocean Trust Mango Martini
Cosmopolitan
Perfect Patron Margarita
Chocolate Martini
Classic Vodka Martini
Bonefish Martini
Espresso Martini
Lemon Drop Martini
Hpnotiq Breeze Martini
Sour Apple Martini

Disclaimer: We do not guarantee, nor do these restaurants guarantee that any menu item will be 100% gluten-free. These restaurants & Business Graphics Group assume no liability for your use of this information. See full disclaimer on page 7.

Boston Market

The following information about gluten-free menu items has been obtained either from the restaurant's website or through direct contact with guest services via email or phone.

This list is compiled based on production information provided by Boston Market approved food manufacturers as of the date published. Boston Market does not guarantee that cross-contact with other gluten-containing products or allergens will not occur. We encourage anyone with food sensitivities, allergies, or special dietary needs to check back on a regular basis for up-to-date information.

Entrees:
Rotisserie Chicken
Roasted Turkey Breast

Sides:
Butternut Squash (regional)
Cinnamon Apples
Creamed Spinach
Fresh Fruit Salad
Fresh Steamed Vegetables
Garlic Dill New Potatoes
Green Beans
Mashed Potatoes
Sweet Corn
Poultry Gravy *(note: Beef Au Jus and Beef Gravy are NOT Gluten-Free)*

Salads: *(no dressing)*
Market Chopped Salad
Market Chopped Salad With Chicken

Corn Bread is NOT Gluten-Free, ask server to leave off the plate.

Disclaimer: We do not guarantee, nor do these restaurants guarantee that any menu item will be 100% gluten-free. These restaurants & Business Graphics Group assume no liability for your use of this information. See full disclaimer on page 7.

Brueggers

The following information about gluten-free menu items has been obtained either from the restaurant's website or through direct contact with guest services via email or phone.

List of Wheat-Free Menu Items (gluten is not listed on their allergen chart): *Note: All of their breads and bagels contain wheat/gluten.*

Beverages:
Brueggaccino
Café au Lait
Café Mocha
Cappuccino
Espresso
Flavored Coffee
French Roast Coffee
House Blend Coffee
Iced Coffee
Hot Teas
Oregon Chai Tea
Hot Chocolate
Almond Flavored Syrup
Chocolate Syrup
Hazelnut Flavored Syrup
Vanilla Flavored Syrup

Cream Cheese:
Bacon Scallion
Cucumber Dill (seasonal)
Garden Veggie
Honey Walnut
Jalapeno
Light Garden Veggie
Light Herb Garlic
Light Plain
Olive Pimiento
Onion and Chive
Plain
Pumpkin (seasonal)
Smoked Salmon
Strawberry Vermont Maple

Salads:
Build Your Own Base
Mandarin Medley/ No Dressing
Mandarin Medley/ Balsamic Vinaigrette

Dressings:
Balsamic Vinaigrette
Ranch

Soups:
Butternut Squash
Fire Roasted Tomato

Misc:
Hummus
All Cheeses
Egg Patties & Omelets
Egg White Patty
Spinach & Cheddar Omelet
Whole Egg Patty

Meat:
Bacon
Ham
Roast Beef
Salmon
Sausage
Turkey
Nuts/Vegetables/Fruits
Almonds (sliced)
Sesame Seeds
Capers
Cucumbers
Green Peppers
Jalapenos
Lettuce
Pickles
Red Onions
Roasted Red Peppers
Sprouts
Tomatoes
Cranberries (dried)
Mandarin Oranges

*Chicken Breast, Chicken Salad and Tuna Salad contain Wheat

Disclaimer: We do not guarantee, nor do these restaurants guarantee that any menu item will be 100% gluten-free. These restaurants & Business Graphics Group assume no liability for your use of this information. See full disclaimer on page 7.

Buca di Beppo

The following information about gluten-free menu items has been obtained either from the restaurant's website or through direct contact with guest services via email or phone.

We would like to make every effort to provide a safe and enjoyable dining experience for our allergic and sensitive guests. Please find attached a list of our gluten-free options. At this time, we cannot prepare gluten-free pasta in our kitchen because of the presence of wheat pasta in the pasta cooker. Due to shared food preparation and cooking areas, it is possible for menu items to inadvertently come into contact with a food allergen from another menu item or food preparation materials. While we do take great care to try and prevent the presence of allergens in your menu item, we are not able to guarantee that your menu item has not come in contact with potential allergens.

Please speak with a member of our management staff if you have special dietary needs or specific food allergies.

Insalate:
Mixed Green Salad (spice up your salad with prosciutto and Gorgonzola by request)
Apple Gorgonzola Salad
Chopped Antipasto Salad
Mozzarella Caprese

Entrees:
Chicken Cacciatore *(request that this dish not be dusted with flour)*
Chicken Marsala *(request that this dish not be dusted with flour)*
Saltimbocca – Chicken or Veal *(request that this dish not be dusted with flour)*
Chicken Limone *(request that this dish not be dusted with flour)*
Salmon Limone *(request that this dish not be dusted with flour)*

Sides:
Garlic Mashed Potatoes
Italian Broccoli Romano *(request that this dish be made separately)*
Green Beans *(request that this dish be made separately)*
Sausage & Peppers

Disclaimer: We do not guarantee, nor do these restaurants guarantee that any menu item will be 100% gluten-free. These restaurants & Business Graphics Group assume no liability for your use of this information. See full disclaimer on page 7.

Buffalo Wild Wings

The following information about gluten-free menu items has been obtained either from the restaurant's website or through direct contact with guest services via email or phone.

Buffalo Wilds Wings does not have a specific gluten free menu. Attached is our Allergen Reference Sheet, Sauce Nutritional information for your review. Please note the preparation process below for the fried items in regards to the crossover of food.

The Naked chicken tenders do not contain gluten and they are cooked on the grill this may be a great alternative.

Preparation Processes:
- Our Traditional Wings are a fresh chicken product that we deep fry at 350'F and shake in the sauce of choice.
- Our Boneless Wings are a breaded chicken product that is also fried at 350'F and then shook in the sauce of choice. The same container is used to sauce the boneless and the traditional wings.
- Our grilled chicken products and burger products are cooked on a 550'F char broiler, a grill seasoning is applied at the time of cooking the seasoning does contain Dairy and Soy. The Burgers do contain gluten.
- Our Tortilla chips are fried fresh in the restaurant.

As a note, in the preparation process of all our fried items we do not segregate individual product into separate fryers when they are cooked so there is the potential of crossover of fried items and oil in the fryers.

Gluten-Free Menu Items:
Naked Tenders w/ Seasoning
Bleu Cheese Dressing
Ranch Dressing
SW Ranch Dressing
Celery
Coleslaw
Salsa
Ice Cream w/ Chocolate Sauce

Dressings:
Bleu Cheese Dressing
Ranch Dressing
SW Ranch Dressing
Caesar Dressing
BBQ Ranch Dressing
Marinara Sauce
Queso Cheese Sauce
Salsa

Sauces:
Sweet BBQ Wing Sauce
Mild Wing Sauce
Parmesan Garlic Wing Sauce
Medium Wing Sauce
Honey BBQ Wing Sauce
Honey Mustard Dipping Sauce
Spicy Garlic Swing Sauce
Caribbean Jerk Wing Sauce
Hot Wing Sauce
Hot BBQ Wing Sauce
Mango Habanero Wing Sauce
Wild Wing Sauce
Blazin Wing Sauce
SW Chipotle

Disclaimer: We do not guarantee, nor do these restaurants guarantee that any menu item will be 100% gluten-free. These restaurants & Business Graphics Group assume no liability for your use of this information. See full disclaimer on page 7.

Bugaboo Creek Steakhouse

The following information about gluten-free menu items has been obtained either from the restaurant's website or through direct contact with guest services via email or phone.

Gluten Restricted Diet Menu *Although Bugaboo Creek does not have a Gluten Free kitchen, we will make every attempt to meet your Gluten Free needs. Bugaboo Creek Steak House, in cooperation with the Gluten Intolerance Group (www.gluten.net) is currently publishing a Gluten Free menu. The items listed on the Gluten Free menu are gluten free or can be ordered gluten free with minor changes. To ensure that your meal is prepared gluten free, please request that all items are prepared in separate containers and on clean food contact surfaces. Updated April 15, 2009*

The Creek's Salads: *(Request NO croutons on salads. Request that salads are prepared in separate bowl from other salads.)*
Alpine Chicken Salad
Chicken Caesar Salad
Bleu Mountain Steak Salad *(order un-marinated steak only and without onion strings)*

Salad Dressings: Caesar, Thousand Island, Balsamic Vinaigrette, Blue Cheese Dressing, Parmesan Peppercorn and Lite Olive Oil Vinaigrette

Bugaboo Steaks:
Timber Creek T-Bone Steak
Mountain Man Strip
Prime Rib *(order without Au Jus sauce)*
Black Magic Steak
Lodge Center Cut Filet
Kansas City Bone-in NY Strip Steak
Kain's Cast Iron Skillet Steak

Fish from the Grill:
Grilled Rainbow Trout
Daily Fresh Fish Fillet *(order without rice)*

Mountain Outfitters' Specials:
Smoked Baby Back Ribs *(order without french fries)*
Moosebreath Burger *(order without bun or french fries)*
Roasted Half Chicken
Campfire Cheesesteak *(order without bun or french fries)*

Sides:
Charlie's Smashed Potatoes, Fresh Steamed Vegetables, Mountain Loaded Baked Potato *(real bacon only)*, Sautéed Mushrooms, Grilled Onions, Baked Beans

Specialty Drinks: All Moose Juices, Rocky Mountain Mudslide, Glacier Freeze Smoothies, All others

---

Disclaimer: We do not guarantee, nor do these restaurants guarantee that any menu item will be 100% gluten-free. These restaurants & Business Graphics Group assume no liability for your use of this information. See full disclaimer on page 7.

Burger King

The information on the Gluten-Sensitive List is based on suppliers' ingredient lists and is as complete as possible at the time of publication (May 2010). However, actual gluten content of these foods and ingredients may vary, depending on the supplier, product handling, and each restaurant's food preparation practices. Burger King Corporation, its franchisees, and employees, do not assume responsibility for a person's sensitivity or allergy to any food item provided in our restaurants. Please always consult your healthcare practitioner for questions regarding your diet. We encourage anyone with food sensitivities, allergies or special dietary needs to communicate any specific food handling requirements to the server or restaurant manager and to check www.bk.com on a regular basis to obtain the most up-to-date information about our food before you order.

BK Positive Steps® Gluten-Sensitive List: Foods and ingredients without wheat, barley, oats or rye. *Actual gluten content may vary depending upon the supplier, product handling, and each restaurant's food preparation practices.*

Meats, Eggs and Sides:
Whopper® Patty
Whopper JR. ® Patty
Steakhouse XT ™Patty
Hamburger Patty
BK BURGER SHOTS ® Patty
Bacon Slice
Ham Slice
TENDERGRILL ® Chicken Breast Filet
Egg Omelet
Southwest Potato Mix
Liquid Eggs
Tacos * *(may be fried with gluten-containing foods)*
French Fries * *(may be fried with gluten-containing foods)*
Sausage Patty * *(may be fried with gluten containing foods)*

Condiments:
Breakfast syrup
Grape Jam
Honey
Ketchup
Mustard
Mayonnaise
Strawberry Jam
Sliced Pickles

Dairy:
Processed American Cheese
Processed Pepper Jack Cheese
Processed Cheddar (Sharp)
Processed Swiss Cheese
Three Cheese Blend
Fat-Free Milk
1% Low fat Chocolate Milk
Chocolate, Vanilla and Strawberry Shakes
Soft-Serve in a cup

Produce:
BK® Fresh Apple Fries
Lettuce
Sliced Onions
Carrots
Sliced Tomato
Salad Mix

Beverages:
Barq's ® Root Beer
Frozen Coca-Cola® Classic
Coca-Cola ® Classic
Coca-Cola ®, Diet Coke ®
Dr. Pepper ®
Sprite ®
Minute Maid ® Lemonade
Minute Maid ® 100% Apple and Orange Juice
Coffees

Disclaimer: We do not guarantee, nor do these restaurants guarantee that any menu item will be 100% gluten-free. These restaurants & Business Graphics Group assume no liability for your use of this information. See full disclaimer on page 7.

Burger King Continued:

Sauces, Dips, Dressings:
BBQ Dipping Sauce
Buffalo Dipping Sauce
Stacker Sauce
Smoky Cheese Sauce
Caramel Sauce
Chocolate Fudge sauce
Sweet and Sour Dipping Sauce
French Fry Sauce
Honey Mustard Dipping Sauce
Marinara Sauce
Ranch Dipping sauce
A1® Thick and Hearty Steak sauce
Sweet Baby Ray's Hot 'n Spicy BBQ Sauce
Tartar Sauce
Zesty Onion Ring Sauce
Vanilla Icing
KEN'S ® Honey Mustard, Light Italian, Ranch

Disclaimer: We do not guarantee, nor do these restaurants guarantee that any menu item will be 100% gluten-free. These restaurants & Business Graphics Group assume no liability for your use of this information. See full disclaimer on page 7.

Burtons Grill

Gluten Free Menu Sample: *Many of Burtons menu items are naturally gluten-free. The selection in this menu is a combination of those items, and items that have been modified to meet the gluten-free criteria. Modified items are indicated in teal. Please let your server know that you are gluten-intolerant so that our chefs take extra care in preparing your meal.*

Appetizers: Grilled Stuffed Zucchini | Calamari | Sesame Crusted Tuna

Salads :
House Salad
Wedge Salad
Caesar Salad
Mediterranean Salad
Barbeque Chicken Salad
Cobb Salad

Sandwiches & Burgers: served on a gluten free bun – fries are gluten free
Classic Cheese Burger
Burtons Burger
Haddock Sandwich
Steak Sandwich
Fish Sandwich

Sides: seasonal vegetable | hand cut french fries | cole slaw

Desserts: Sorbet | Vanilla Bean Creme Brulee | Warmed Chocolate Torte | Vanilla Ice Cream

Chef Specials:
Risotto of the Day
Salmon Picatta
Jambalaya
Chicken Salad Plate

Fresh Seafood:
Salmon
Scallops

Entrees and Steaks:
Tuscan Brick Chicken
Ribeye
New York Strip
Chicken & Mushroom Pasta**
prepared with fresh gluten free pasta, please allow additional time for preparation

Please note: If you have specific dietary requirements, allergies or preferences, please ask your server for details. In Partnership with the Gluten-Free Restaurant Awareness Program® a Program of the Gluten intolerance Group®. For more information visit www.glutenfreerestaurants.org

Locations:
94 Derby Street, Suite 279, Hingham, MA, 02043
145 Turnpike Street, North Andover, MA, 01845
1363 Boylston Street, Boston, MA, 02215
100 Evergreen Way, South Windsor, CT 06074
741 First Colonial Road, Virginia Beach, VA, 23451

Disclaimer: We do not guarantee, nor do these restaurants guarantee that any menu item will be 100% gluten-free. These restaurants & Business Graphics Group assume no liability for your use of this information. See full disclaimer on page 7.

California Pizza Kitchen

The following information about gluten-free menu items has been obtained either from the restaurant's website or through direct contact with guest services via email or phone.

Please be advised, the majority of menu items served at California Pizza Kitchen contain gluten. In addition, the majority of our salad dressings also contain gluten.

It would be safe for you to order the:

Field Greens Salad with Gorgonzola
Grilled Vegetable Salad
House Salad with *no croutons or Steamed Vegetables*
Dijon Balsamic Vinaigrette Salad Dressing
Olive Oil is also available upon request.

These are just a few suggestions. If you have specific questions, please ask your server when you place your order.

As California Pizza Kitchen serves many items that do contain gluten, please be aware that it is not possible to guarantee that cross contamination will not occur.

Disclaimer: We do not guarantee, nor do these restaurants guarantee that any menu item will be 100% gluten-free. These restaurants & Business Graphics Group assume no liability for your use of this information. See full disclaimer on page 7.

The Capital Grille

The following information about gluten-free menu items has been obtained either from the restaurant's website or through direct contact with guest services via email or phone.

Please notify the Chef or a manager upon arrival and we will use new tongs and pans to prepare your food and take extra steps to keep your food away from items with gluten. While we do have flour in our kitchens, and as such, cannot guarantee a gluten free experience, the items listed below are made from recipes that do not include gluten.

Appetizers:
Wagyu Carpaccio
Oysters on the half shell *ordered without mignonette sauce*
Shrimp Cocktail
Cold Shellfish Platter *ordered without mignonette sauce*

Salads:
Caesar Salad *ordered without croutons*
Garden Salad *ordered without dressing*
The Wedge Salad *ordered without dressing*
Spinach Salad *ordered without dressing*

Entrees:
Any steak *ordered without sauce*
Lamb Chops
Veal Chop *ordered without sauce*
Fresh Lobster
Fresh Seared Salmon fillet *ordered without citrus glaze*
Fresh Swordfish Jardinière
Sesame Seared Tuna *ordered without ginger vinegar and without white soy*
Roasted Chicken

Dessert:
Crème Brulée
Fresh Berries with Vanilla Cream
Sorbet
Flourless Chocolate Espresso Cake

Disclaimer: We do not guarantee, nor do these restaurants guarantee that any menu item will be 100% gluten-free. These restaurants & Business Graphics Group assume no liability for your use of this information. See full disclaimer on page 7.

Captain D's Seafood Kitchen

The following information about gluten-free menu items has been obtained either from the restaurant's website or through direct contact with guest services via email or phone.

Our products may contain one or more allergens, including fish, shellfish, wheat, soy, soy derivatives, milk and eggs. Our products generally do not contain peanuts or tree nuts but may come from manufacturing equipment used in common with those nuts. In addition, we prepare our products in and on common restaurant equipment and, therefore, our products may contain allergens not specific to the products being ordered.

Fish:
Catfish
Wild Alaskan Salmon
Seasoned Tilapia Dinner

Shrimp:
Premium Shrimp
Scampi Shrimp
Shrimp Skewers

Salads:
Wild Alaskan Salmon Salad

Sides:
Baked Potato – *Plain*
Side Salad
Roasted Red Potatoes
Corn on the Cob
Broccoli

Sauces:
Ginger Teriyaki Sauce
Scampi Butter Sauce
Sweet Chili Sauce
Tartar Sauce
Cocktail Sauce
Ranch Dressing
Blue Cheese Dressing
Honey Mustard Dressing

Disclaimer: We do not guarantee, nor do these restaurants guarantee that any menu item will be 100% gluten-free. These restaurants & Business Graphics Group assume no liability for your use of this information. See full disclaimer on page 7.

Carino's Italian Restaurant

The following information about gluten-free menu items has been obtained either from the restaurant's website or through direct contact with guest services via email or phone.

Important: *It is important to let your server know the specific modifications for each of your menu selections. If you have any questions, please ask to speak with a manager. This menu and the information on it are provided by Carino's Italian, in cooperation with the Gluten Intolerance Group (GIG), as a service to our guests. Carino's Italian and GIG assume no responsibility for its use and information. Guests are encouraged to consider this information in light of their individual requirements and needs.*

Appetizers and Salads:

Shrimp Scampi (*Order without garlic toast*)
House Salad (*Order without croutons*)
Caesar Salad (*Order without croutons*)
Italian Wedge

Dressing Choices: House Chianti Vinaigrette, Creamy Gorgonzola, Ranch, Roasted Garlic Ranch, Signature Caesar, Sundried Tomato Balsamic Vinaigrette

Soups:
Italian Chili
Roasted Garlic Potato Soup (*Order without croutons*)

Entrees:
Lemon Rosemary Chicken (*Substitute garlic sautéed spinach, potatoes or extra green beans or vegetables instead of pasta*)
Jalapeno Garlic Tilapia (*Order without flour on the tilapia. Substitute sautéed green beans, garlic sautéed spinach or potatoes instead of pasta*)
Chicken Scaloppini (*Order without flour on the chicken. Substitute sautéed green beans, garlic sautéed spinach or potatoes instead of pasta*)
Chicken Marsala (*Order without flour on the chicken. Substitute sautéed green beans, garlic sautéed spinach or potatoes instead of pasta*)
Grilled Citrus Balsamic Salmon (*Substitute sautéed green beans, extra garlic sautéed spinach or potatoes instead of pasta*)
Italian Pot Roast (*Order with potatoes*)

Kid's Menu:
Kid's Grilled Chicken (*Substitute sautéed green beans or potatoes instead of pasta*)

Dessert:
Vanilla Ice Cream With chocolate syrup, caramel sauce or amarena cherries.

Disclaimer: We do not guarantee, nor do these restaurants guarantee that any menu item will be 100% gluten-free. These restaurants & Business Graphics Group assume no liability for your use of this information. See full disclaimer on page 7.

Carl's Jr

The following information about gluten-free menu items has been obtained either from the restaurant's website or through direct contact with guest services via email or phone.

The information contained on this chart is based on standard U.S. product formulations. Variations may occur due to a variety of factors and circumstances, including, but not limited to differences in suppliers, ingredient substitutions, recipe revisions, product assembly and seasonal variances. Product participation may vary by location and test products are not included. This information is current as of April 1, 2009. The information on this chart is reported for informational purposes only by Carl Karcher Enterprises, Inc. Neither CKE, its franchisees, or its employees assume any responsibility for sensitivity or allergy to any food product provided in our restaurants. Anyone with food sensitivities, allergies, or special dietary needs should consult a medical professional regarding the suitability of our food products, and should regularly review the information contained at www. Carlsjr.com for content updates. If you have specific questions about our menu, call 1-877-799-STAR.

List of Wheat-Free Menu Items (gluten is not listed on their allergen chart):

Burgers and Sides:
The Low Carb Six Dollar Burger
Natural Cut Fries *(ask if fries are prepared in a dedicated fryer)*
Chili Cheese Fries *(ask if fries are prepared in a dedicated fryer)*

Salads and Dressings:
Side Salad
House Dressing
Blue Cheese Dressing
Thousand Island Dressing
Low Fat Balsamic Dressing

Dessert:
Vanilla Shake
Chocolate Shake
Strawberry Shake

Disclaimer: We do not guarantee, nor do these restaurants guarantee that any menu item will be 100% gluten-free. These restaurants & Business Graphics Group assume no liability for your use of this information. See full disclaimer on page 7.

Carrabbas

This menu and the information on it are provided by Carrabba's Italian Grill, in cooperation with the Gluten intolerance Group ("GIG"), as a service to our customers. Carrabba's and GIG assume no responsibility for its use and any resulting liability or consequential damages are denied. Cynthia Kupper, a Registered Dietitian with GIG, prepared this information (which has not been verified by Carrabba's.) Our management teams and service staff are not trained on the intricacies of Celiac Disease or gluten intolerance and cannot be expected to provide recommendations or other advice on this issue. All questions and requests for recommendations should be directed to GIG or the Carrabba's corporate office. Patrons are encouraged to consider the information provided, to their own satisfaction, in light of their individual needs and requirements.

Antipasti: Cozze in Bianco or Shrimp Scampi – *request no garlic toast*

Zuppe:
Mama Mandola's Sicilian Chicken Soup – *Request no pasta be added*

Insalate: All Salads – *Request no croutons and to be mixed in a fresh bowl*
Insalada Carrabba – *Request the chicken to be made without grill baste*
Insalata Carrabba Caesar – *Request the chicken/shrimp to be made without grill baste*
Insalata Johnny Rocco – *Request the seafood to be made without grill baste*
Insalata Fiorucci
House Salads: House, Italian, Caesar or Mediterranean Salad

*Many of our meats are cooked on the same grill. We do not have a gluten-free grill. *All grill items: request to be made without grill baste.*

Family Classics & Combinations:
The Johnny, Chicken Trio or The Carrabba

Marsala: Chicken, Sirloin or Pork Chops

Wood Burning Grill:
Chicken Bryan, Ollo Rosa Maria, Chicken Gratella, Filet Fiorentina or Norwegian Salmon

Gluten free fish sauces: Bellimbusto, Citriolini, Denisco, Ferre, Lemon Butter, Tri-Bell Pepper, Livornese, Mostarda, Nocciola, Nino, Positano, Roasted Tomato Salsa di Pepperoni, Salsa Verde, Sundried Tomato Pesto, Tomato Basil, Vinaigrette

Bambini Menu:
Grilled Chicken Breast – *Request the chicken to be made without grill baste*

Dolci: John Cole - Blue Bell vanilla ice cream with caramel sauce and roasted cinnamon rum pecans

---

Disclaimer: We do not guarantee, nor do these restaurants guarantee that any menu item will be 100% gluten-free. These restaurants & Business Graphics Group assume no liability for your use of this information. See full disclaimer on page 7.

Charley's Grilled Subs

The following information about gluten-free menu items has been obtained either from the restaurant's website or through direct contact with guest services via email or phone.

All nutritional information is based on data from Charley's approved suppliers and manufacturers. Variations in distributors, product substitutions, procedural changes, portioning, seasonality and manufacturers may alter the actual nutritional values listed. Questions & Comments: Contact R & D Department at 614-923-4700

List of Wheat-Free Menu Items (gluten is not listed on their allergen chart):

Breakfast:
Two Eggs Scrambled
Ham Omelet
Bacon Omelet
Sausage Omelet
Veggie Omelet
Western Omelet
Hash Browns (*check to see if they are fried with other gluten-containing items*)

Salads:
Grilled Chicken Salad
Chicken Teriyaki Salad
Buffalo Chicken Salad
Grilled Steak Salad
Fresh Garden Salad

Dressing:
Ranch Dressing
Italian Dressing

Disclaimer: We do not guarantee, nor do these restaurants guarantee that any menu item will be 100% gluten-free. These restaurants & Business Graphics Group assume no liability for your use of this information. See full disclaimer on page 7.

Charlie Brown's Steakhouse

The following information about gluten-free menu items has been obtained either from the restaurant's website or through direct contact with guest services via email or phone.

The following has been analyzed by an independent registered dietician and is meant to serve as a guide to help choose items they have deemed to be gluten free. Charlie Brown's is not responsible for the content based on the dietician's recommendations.

Sauces, side dishes, starches or any other condiment, unless otherwise listed on this menu, should be presumed to contain gluten. Only the items listed have been analyzed and are separate from any side dishes or sauces that may normally accompany each entrée.

Appetizers:
Grilled Shrimp (*no bread, sauce or frizzled onions*)

Salads/Soups:
Caesar Salad (*without croutons*)
Chicken Caesar (*without croutons*)
Steakhouse Wedge Salad
French Onion Soup (*no bread*)

Entrees: *All steaks would have to be untopped and with no frizzled onions*
NY Strip*
Chopped Steak*
Filet Mignon*
Porterhouse*
Top Sirloin*
Prime Rib*
Tilapia (*no lemon butter sauce*)
Flounder (*simply broiled*)
Salmon (*not marinated, no sauce*)
Roast Chicken (*no sauce*)
Rack of Lamb (*no crust or garlic aioli*, demi glace is ok)
BBQ Ribs
Twin Tails

Sandwiches:
Chicken salad (*no bread*)
Hibachi Chicken Sandwich (*no bread*)
All Burgers (*no bread*)

Sauces/Condiments:
Au Jus
Barbecue Sauce
Buffalo Wing Sauce
Cocktail Sauce
Guacamole
Honey Mustard Sauce
Ketchup
Marinara Sauce
Mayonnaise
Melted Butter
Mustard
Orange Horseradish Sauce
Salsa
Sour Cream
Sour Cream Horseradish Sauce
Steak Sauce, A-1
Tomato Basil Bruschetta
All Salad Dressings (*except Asian and Ranch*)

Vegetables/Sides:
Garlic mashed potatoes
Fresh steamed broccoli
Baked potato
Sautéed onions
Seasoned rice
Roasted vegetable medley
Fresh steamed asparagus
Sherried button mushrooms
Sweet potato mashed
Coleslaw

Disclaimer: We do not guarantee, nor do these restaurants guarantee that any menu item will be 100% gluten-free. These restaurants & Business Graphics Group assume no liability for your use of this information. See full disclaimer on page 7.

Cheeseburger in Paradise

We are proud to offer a full gluten-free menu to accommodate our customers. Menu items should be ordered as suggested. This menu and the information on it are provided by Cheeseburger in Paradise, in cooperation with the Gluten Intolerance Group (GIG), as a service to our customers. For more information on Gluten, please visit www.gluten.net

Appetizers:
Mini-Cheeseburgers *(ORDER WITHOUT BUNS)*

Soups & Salads:
Choice of dressings include: Citrus Vinaigrette, Coconut Curry, Spicy Ranch, Balsamic Vinaigrette, Honey Mustard and Buffalo Blue Cheese.
Calypso Chicken Salad *Substitute blackened shrimp*
Son of a Sailor Salad *(ORDER WITHOUT WONTONS)*
Costa Rican Steak Salad *(ORDER WITHOUT WONTONS)*

Burgers: *(ORDER WITHOUT BUN)*
Bacon Cheddar Burger
BBQ Cheddar Burger *(without Fried Onion Strings)*
Mushroom Swiss Burger
Baja Burger
Cheeseburger In Paradise Burger
Mini-Cheeseburgers
Veggie Burger

Island Specialties:
Parrot Beach Salmon *(ORDER GRILLED OR BLACKENED WITHOUT SAUCE, ISLAND RICE OR TERIYAKI BROCCOLI)*
BBQ Ribs
St. Barts Citrus Chicken *(ORDER WITHOUT ISLAND RICE OR TERIYAKI BROCCOLI)*

Sandwiches: *(ORDER WITHOUT BUN AND SWEET POTATO CHIPS)*
Bayside BBQ Chicken Sandwich
Caribbean Chicken Sandwich
Mahi Mahi Sandwich

Kid's Menu
For children under 10. Includes beverage and a choice of side.
Mini-Cheeseburgers *(ORDER WITHOUT BUN)*
Grilled Chicken Breast
Lil' Pirates Treat *(ORDER WITHOUT OREO® COOKIE CRUMBLES)*

Sensuous Treat:
Copa Banana *(ORDER WITHOUT NILLA WAFERS)*

Sides:
Coleslaw
French Fried Potatoes
Vegetable of the Day *(ORDER WITHOUT ROASTED GARLIC BUTTER)*

Beverages:
Cheeseburger in Paradise Cocktail
Island Paradise
Blueberry Mojito
Blackberry Sangria
Tranquil Breeze
Silver Sunset
Surfside Sodas
Mouth-Watering Milkshakes
Jamaican Root Beer Float
Island Lemonade
Strawberry Lemonade
Flavored Iced Tea (Peach, Mango, Pomegranate, Raspberry and Blueberry)
Bottled Water
Red Bull
Freshly Brewed Iced Tea
Freshly Brewed Coffee
Sodas: Coke, Diet Coke, Sprite, Barq's Root Beer, Orange, Fresca.

Disclaimer: We do not guarantee, nor do these restaurants guarantee that any menu item will be 100% gluten-free. These restaurants & Business Graphics Group assume no liability for your use of this information. See full disclaimer on page 7.

Cheeseburger in Paradise Continued:

This menu and the information on it are provided by Cheeseburger in Paradise, in cooperation with the Gluten Intolerance Group (GIG), as a service to our customers. Cheeseburger in Paradise and GIG assume no responsibility for its use and any resulting liability or consequential damages are denied. Cynthia Kupper, a Registered Dietician with GIG, prepared this information (which has not been verified by Cheeseburger in Paradise). Our management teams and service staff are not trained on the intricacies of Celiac Disease or gluten intolerance and cannot be expected to provide recommendations or other advice on this issue. All questions should be directed to GIG or the Cheeseburger in Paradise home office. Patrons are encouraged to consider the information provided, to their own satisfaction and individual needs and requirements. *For more information on gluten please visit www.gluten.net*

Disclaimer: We do not guarantee, nor do these restaurants guarantee that any menu item will be 100% gluten-free. These restaurants & Business Graphics Group assume no liability for your use of this information. See full disclaimer on page 7.

Cheesecake Factory

The following information about gluten-free menu items has been obtained either from the restaurant's website or through direct contact with guest services via email or phone.

Although we prepare dishes that we do not add wheat, oats, rye or barley, our concern is that some of our sub-ingredients may contain trace amounts of gluten, particularly imported ingredients.

Because we understand that sensitivities can vary, our managers will be happy to help you select dishes to which we do not add wheat, oats, rye or barley. Our servers and managers are extremely knowledgeable about all the ingredients in our dishes. Under the strictest guidelines, we recommend non-marinated vegetables, chicken, steak, shrimp or fish, pan cooked as opposed to grilled.

We do have one cheesecake that we serve in our restaurants that is made without any flour or wheat, which is our Godiva Chocolate Cheesecake. I do want to mention that it is baked, cooled and stored in the same facility with all of our cheesecakes, so we cannot guarantee against unintentional cross-contamination.

Our kitchen operations team is currently working on a list of gluten free menu items to make dining in our restaurants easier for our guests with dietary restrictions.

Disclaimer: We do not guarantee, nor do these restaurants guarantee that any menu item will be 100% gluten-free. These restaurants & Business Graphics Group assume no liability for your use of this information. See full disclaimer on page 7.

Chick-Fil-A

The following information about gluten-free menu items has been obtained either from the restaurant's website or through direct contact with guest services via email or phone.

The following Information is for customers who have intolerance to gluten (wheat, barley, rye, triticale, oats, and spelt). Chick-fil-A menu items listed below may fit your gluten diet. This information was obtained from the suppliers of each of the items. We have bolded the grain source on items where customers have had questions. Some ingredients such as spices and natural flavors may be proprietary; therefore, we may not have the source listed for those items. We recommend you review this list with your physician before consuming any of the products listed below, or any other item on our menu. An ingredient list for all of these items can be found at: http://www.chick-fil-a.com/Documents/GlutenFreeItemsList.pdf

Entrées:
Chick-fil-A® Chargrilled Chicken Sandwich filet *(no bun)*
Chick-fil-A® Chargrilled Chicken Garden Salad
Chick-fil-A® Chargrilled Chicken & Fruit Salad
Tortilla Strips

Sides:
Fruit Cup
Side Salad
Cole Slaw
Carrot & Raisin Salad
Chick-fil-A® Waffle Potato Fries ® *(confirm that they are cooked in separate fryers from the chicken)*
Yogurt Parfait

Breakfast:
Bacon Slice
Egg
Sausage Patty
American Cheese Slice
Hash Browns (available for breakfast only) *(confirm that they are cooked in separate fryers from the chicken)*

Desserts:
Icedream®
Chocolate Syrup
Blueberry Topping

Beverages:
All beverages

Dipping Sauces and Dressings:
Barbeque Sauce
Honey Mustard Sauce
Honey Roasted BBQ Sauce
Polynesian Sauce
Buttermilk Ranch Sauce
Chick-fil-A® Buffalo Sauce
Spicy Dressing
Blue Cheese Dressing
Buttermilk Ranch Dressing
Thousand Island Dressing
Light Italian Dressing
Fat Free Dijon Honey Mustard Dressing
Caesar Dressing
Reduced Fat Raspberry Vinaigrette Dressing
Reduced Fat Berry Balsamic Vinaigrette Dressing
Chick-fil-A® Sauce

Condiments:
Ketchup
Mustard Mayonnaise
Apple Jelly
Grape Jelly
Mixed Fruit Jelly

Disclaimer: We do not guarantee, nor do these restaurants guarantee that any menu item will be 100% gluten-free. These restaurants & Business Graphics Group assume no liability for your use of this information. See full disclaimer on page 7.

Chili's

Suggested Beverage & Menu Options for WHEAT/GLUTEN Allergies: We have prepared this suggested list of beverage and menu options based on the most current ingredient information from our food suppliers and their stated absence of wheat/gluten within these items. Please be aware that during normal kitchen operations involving shared cooking and preparation areas, including common fryer oil, the possibility exists for food items to come in contact with other food products. <u>Due to these circumstances, we are unable to guarantee that any menu entrée can be completely free of allergens.</u> PRIOR TO PLACING YOUR ORDER, PLEASE ALWAYS ALERT THE MANAGER TO YOUR FOOD ALLERGY OR SPECIAL DIETARY NEEDS.

Soups:
Chicken & Green Chile
Sweet Corn

Salads:
(Without Dressing & Croutons & Tortilla Strips)
Grilled BBQ Chicken Salad
Caribbean Salad: Chicken option ONLY w/ honey Lime Dressing
Chicken Caesar Salad
House Salad

Salad Dressings:
Citrus Balsamic Vinaigrette
Honey Lime
Honey Mustard

Slow Smoked In-House Ribs:
Original *(without sides)*

Everything's Better on the Grill:
(Listed w/o Condiments & Sides Unless Indicated)
Classic Sirloin *w/o Garlic Toast*
Flame Grilled Ribeye *w/o Garlic Toast*
GG Salmon w/ Rice & Veggies
GG Sirloin w/ Veggies
Grilled Salmon w/ Garlic & Herbs w/ Rice & Veggies
Margarita Chicken w/ Rice & Black Beans *w/o Tortilla Strips*
Monterey Chicken w/ Mashed Potatoes *w/o Gravy & Veggies*

Pepper Pals:
(All Listed w/o Bun & Fires & O Strings)
Grilled Chicken Platter
Grilled Chicken Sandwich
Little Mouth Cheeseburger

Burgers:
(All Listed w/o Bun & Fries & O Strings)
Bacon Burger
Ground Peppercorn Burger w/o Bleu Cheese Dressing
Mushroom-Swiss Burger
Old-timer Burger

Sides:
Black Beans
Corn on the Cob
Seasonal Veggies
Mandarin Oranges
Loaded Mashed Potatoes
Mashed Potatoes *WITHOUT gravy*
Rice

Sauces & Extras:
Avocado Slices
Bacon
Guacamole
Mixed Cheese
Original BBQ Sauce
Pico de Gallo
Salsa
Sautéed Mushrooms

Stupendously Sweet Endings:
Chocolate Shake

Disclaimer: We do not guarantee, nor do these restaurants guarantee that any menu item will be 100% gluten-free. These restaurants & Business Graphics Group assume no liability for your use of this information. See full disclaimer on page 7.

Chili's Continued:

Beverages:
Coke, Dasani Water, Diet Coke, Dr. Pepper, Electric Blue Blast, IBC Root Beer, Rockin' Tropical Punch, Sprite, Strawberry Lemonade, Tea: Blackberry & mango, Red & White Wine.

At Chili's, a top priority is always the health and safety of our guests. As part of our commitment to you, our allergen menus are based on product information provided by Chili's approved food manufacturers. Every effort is made to keep this information current. However, it is possible that ingredient changes and substitutions may occur due to the differences in regional suppliers, recipe revisions, preparation techniques, and/or the season of the year. Certain menu items may vary from restaurant to restaurant and may not be available at all locations. We highly recommend that our guests with food allergies or special dietary needs consult with a restaurant manager prior to placing an order to ensure the posted information is accurate and represents the menu items sold at that particular location. Limited time offers, test products, or regional items have not been included in the menus.

Disclaimer: We do not guarantee, nor do these restaurants guarantee that any menu item will be 100% gluten-free. These restaurants & Business Graphics Group assume no liability for your use of this information. See full disclaimer on page 7.

Chipotle

The following information about gluten-free menu items has been obtained either from the restaurant's website or through direct contact with guest services via email or phone.

Most people wanting to avoid gluten can eat anything we serve except for our burrito tortillas, our soft taco tortillas, and possibly our hot red tomatillo salsa (there is a small amount of distilled vinegar in it which some gluten-oriented websites still say might be problematic, although most don't).

Everything else is fine to eat for most people wanting to avoid gluten, including our crispy corn tacos, our corn chips, and our burrito bowls (no tortilla). However, you should know that it's possible our corn may have a small amount of gluten from potentially co-mingling with gluten-containing grains in the field.

If you are highly sensitive and would like us to change our gloves, we would be happy to do that at your request. Additionally, because our folks work with wheat tortillas all day long, there may be the possibility of cross-contact in our restaurants. We encourage you to carefully consider your dining choices.

From: http://www.chipotle.com/Chipotle_Allergen_Card.pdf

Gluten Free Menu Items:

Barbacoa
Black Beans
Cheese
Chips
Crispy Taco Shells
Chicken
Pinto Beans
Rice
Sour Cream
Steak

"Variations may occur due to differences in suppliers, ingredient substitutions, recipe revisions and/or food preparation at the restaurant. For general information on food allergens, visit the Food Allergy and Anaphylaxis Network Website at http://www.foodallergy.org."

Disclaimer: We do not guarantee, nor do these restaurants guarantee that any menu item will be 100% gluten-free. These restaurants & Business Graphics Group assume no liability for your use of this information. See full disclaimer on page 7.

Claim Jumper

The following information about gluten-free menu items has been obtained either from the restaurant's website or through direct contact with guest services via email or phone.

Gluten Free: *Please specify GLUTEN-FREE when ordering from this menu. These menu items have been modified to be gluten-free. Please be aware that Claim Jumper Restaurants is not a gluten-free establishment and therefore, cross contamination may occur.*

Salads:
Citrus Chicken Salad: *Decline bread choice and no bleu cheese crumbles*
Chicken Caesar Salad: *Decline bread choice and no croutons*

Entrees:
Giant Stuffed Baker
Rotisserie Chicken: *Decline bread choice*
Roasted Tri-Tip: *Decline bread choice and no herb gravy*

Aged Steaks & Lobster: *Decline bread choice*
Certified USDA Prime Top Sirloin
Filet Mignon
Ribeye Steak
New York Steak
Porterhouse Steak
Two steaks in one
Filet Mignon & Lobster Tail
Lobster Tail Dinner
Premium 8oz lobster tail
Prime Rib

Disclaimer: We do not guarantee, nor do these restaurants guarantee that any menu item will be 100% gluten-free. These restaurants & Business Graphics Group assume no liability for your use of this information. See full disclaimer on page 7.

The Coffee Bean and Tea Leaf

The following information about gluten-free menu items has been obtained either from the restaurant's website or through direct contact with guest services via email or phone.

Currently all of our Teas and Coffees are all made with gluten-free ingredients.

Also, currently none of our powders (Vanilla, Chocolate, NSA Vanilla, NSA Chocolate, Hazelnut, etc) contain gluten.

Do know, however, that there may be a possibility of cross contamination while the powders are being produced.

Disclaimer: We do not guarantee, nor do these restaurants guarantee that any menu item will be 100% gluten-free. These restaurants & Business Graphics Group assume no liability for your use of this information. See full disclaimer on page 7.

Cold Stone Creamery

Cake Batter, Cinnamon Bun, Cookie Dough, and Oatmeal Cookie Batter ice creams contain gluten. In addition, any candies that have a flour component to them also contain gluten. Although we take precautions by cleaning the mixing stone often, we cannot guarantee that residual products containing gluten will not accidentally be mixed into your ice cream.

Ice Cream:
- Amaretto
- Banana
- Black Cherry
- Butter Pecan
- Candy Cane
- Chocolate
- Chocolate Raspberry Truffle
- Cinnamon
- Coconut
- Coffee
- Cotton Candy
- Dark Chocolate
- Dark Chocolate Peppermint
- Egg Nog
- French Vanilla
- Ghirardelli
- Irish Cream
- Jello Banana Pudding
- Jello Butterscotch Pudding
- Jello Chocolate Pudding
- Jello Vanilla Pudding
- Macadamia Nut
- Mango
- Marshmallow
- Mint
- Mocha
- Orange Dreamsicle
- Peanut Butter
- Pecan Praline
- Pistachio
- Pumpkin
- Raspberry
- Sinless Sans Fat Sweet Cream
- Strawberry
- Sweet Cream
- Vanilla Bean
- White Chocolate

Sorbet and Yogurt:
- Lemon Sorbet
- Raspberry Sorbet
- Tart and Tangy Yogurt
- Country Time Pink Lemonade Sorbet
- Watermelon Sorbet
- Tart and Tangy Berry Yogurt

Mix-Ins:
- Butterfinger Candy Bar
- Chocolate chips
- Gummi Bears
- Heath Candy Bar
- M&M's Candy
- Reese's Peanut Butter Cup
- Snickers Candy
- White Chocolate Chips
- Almond Joy Candy
- Gumballs
- Peanut M&M's
- Reese's Pieces
- Chocolate Shavings
- York Peppermint Patties
- Coconut
- Marshmallows
- Peanut Butter
- Toasted Coconut

Nuts:
- Macadamia Nuts
- Pecan Pralines
- Pecans
- Roasted Almonds
- Walnuts
- Cashews
- Peanuts
- Pistachio Nuts
- Sliced Almonds

Fruit:
- Apple Pie Filling
- Bananas
- Blackberries
- Black Cherries
- Blueberries
- Cherry Pie Filing
- Maraschino Cherries
- Pineapple Chunks
- Raspberries
- Strawberries
- Peach Pie Filling
- Raisins

Disclaimer: We do not guarantee, nor do these restaurants guarantee that any menu item will be 100% gluten-free. These restaurants & Business Graphics Group assume no liability for your use of this information. See full disclaimer on page 7.

Cold Stone Creamery Continued:

Toppings:

Cinnamon	Whipped Topping	Marshmallow Crème
Honey	Caramel	Butterscotch Fat Free
Rainbow Sprinkles	Fudge	Caramel Fat Free
Redi Wip Original	Chocolate Sprinkles	Fudge Fat Free

Smoothie Products:
Lemon Ice
Mango
Orange Juice
Lifestyle Smoothie Mix
Nrgize Supplement – Protein
Nrgize Supplement – Antioxidant/Immune
Nrgize Supplement – Anti-Stress, Nrgize Supplement – Energy

Disclaimer: We do not guarantee, nor do these restaurants guarantee that any menu item will be 100% gluten-free. These restaurants & Business Graphics Group assume no liability for your use of this information. See full disclaimer on page 7.

Cosi

The following information about gluten-free menu items has been obtained either from the restaurant's website or through direct contact with guest services via email or phone.

Beverages:
Café Au Lait
Cappuccino
Chai Tea Latte
Coffee
Hot Chocolate
Hot Cider
Hot Tea (earl grey, English breakfast, lemon zinger, raspberry zinger, peppermint, green, mandarin orange)
Latte
Mocha
Steamer
Espresso
Espresso Macchiato

Iced Chai Tea Latte
Iced Coffee
Iced Latte
Iced Mocha
Arctic Latte
Arctic Mocha
Strawberry Banana
Mixed Berry
Choc. Cover Straw
Pineapple Mango

Fruit Salad
Omelet

Salad and Soup:
Bombay Chicken Salad
Our Lighter Side Bombay Chicken Salad
Cobb Salad
Our Lighter Side Cobb Salad
Greek Salad
Mixed Green Salad
Salad Bruschetta
Signature Salad
Our Lighter Side Signature Salad
Wild Alaskan Salmon Salad
Tomato Basil Aurora Soup

Dessert:
Frozen Yogurt
Ice Cream Sundae
Ice Cream Scoop
Whipped Cream

Disclaimer: We do not guarantee, nor do these restaurants guarantee that any menu item will be 100% gluten-free. These restaurants & Business Graphics Group assume no liability for your use of this information. See full disclaimer on page 7.

Cracker Barrel Old Country Store

The following information about gluten-free menu items has been obtained either from the restaurant's website or through direct contact with guest services via email or phone.

The following is a list of menu items that do not contain wheat, barley, or rye products as an ingredient (the modified food starch in the fried apples is from corn). However, we have an open kitchen where biscuits and dumplings are made from scratch several times daily. Many of our grill items do not contain glutens but are prepared on the same equipment as products that do. There is always a chance that cross-transference may occur.

Please inform a manager of your sensitivity when you visit one of our stores to ensure that every effort is made to prevent the accidental transfer of glutens via the handling and preparation of your meal.

Grill Items: grilled chicken tenders, hamburger steak, ribeye and sirloin steak, grilled catfish, grilled trout, grilled pork chops, country ham, city ham, bacon, eggs, pork sausage, turkey sausage

Side Items: carrots, cole slaw, corn, fried apples, green beans, mashed potatoes, baked potato, pinto beans, turnip greens

Excluding the fried chicken tender salad and chunky chicken (homemade chicken salad) salad, salads ordered without croutons would not contain glutens. See the ingredient statements below for our salad dressings choice.

The vinegars used in the salad refined distilled grain vinegars. According to the American Celiac Disease Alliance, "Distilled alcoholic beverages and vinegars are gluten-free. Distilled products do not contain any harmful gluten peptides. Research indicates that the gluten peptide is too large to carry over in the distillation process. This leaves the resultant liquid gluten-free."

Buttermilk Dressing: cultured buttermilk, soybean oil, water, egg yolk, distilled vinegar, salt, corn syrup, sugar, spices, lactic acid, xanthan gum, guar gum, onion*, potassium sorbate and sodium benzoate added as preservatives, garlic*, disodium inosinate, disodium guanylate, calcium disodium EDTA added to protect flavor. *DEHYDRATED

Peppercorn Dressing: soybean oil, water, sour cream solids, egg yolk, distilled vinegar, salt, spices, dehydrated garlic, xanthan gum, potassium sorbate and sodium benzoate added as preservatives, natural flavor, calcium disodium EDTA added to protect flavor.

Honey French Dressing: high fructose corn syrup, soybean oil, corn-cider vinegar, distilled vinegar, tomato paste, salt, paprika, spices, xanthan gum, onion*, honey, invert sugar, beet juice concentrate, garlic*, natural flavor. *DEHYDRATED

Disclaimer: We do not guarantee, nor do these restaurants guarantee that any menu item will be 100% gluten-free. These restaurants & Business Graphics Group assume no liability for your use of this information. See full disclaimer on page 7.

Cracker Barrel Continued:

Honey Mustard Dressing: soybean oil, water, high fructose corn syrup, distilled vinegar, honey, egg yolk, mustard seed, sugar, salt, spice, white wine, natural flavor, xanthan gum, citric acid, tartartic acid, artificial color (including yellow #5), calcium disodium EDTA added to protect flavor.

1000 Island Dressing: soybean oil, water, pickles, sugar, tomato paste, distilled vinegar, high fructose corn syrup, egg yolk, salt, spice, sodium benzoate, and potassium sorbate added as preservatives, natural and artificial flavors, onion*, bell peppers, garlic*, calcium disodium EDTA to protect flavor, xanthan gum, guar gum, polysorbate 80. *DEHYDRATED

Disclaimer: We do not guarantee, nor do these restaurants guarantee that any menu item will be 100% gluten-free. These restaurants & Business Graphics Group assume no liability for your use of this information. See full disclaimer on page 7.

Culver's

The following information about gluten-free menu items has been obtained either from the restaurant's website or through direct contact with guest services via email or phone.

Salads:
Chicken Cashew Salad with Flame Roasted
Strawberry Fields Salad

Sides:
Cole Slaw
Green Beans

Soups: (vary by location)
Baja Chicken Enchilada
Mushroom Medley
Potato Au Gratin

Custards:
Chocolate Dish
Chocolate Frozen Custard One Pint
Chocolate Frozen Custard One Quart
Vanilla Dish
Vanilla Frozen Custard One Pint
Vanilla Frozen Custard One Quart

Salad Dressings:
Bleu Cheese Fancy Chunky
Caesar Dressing
French
French Reduced Calorie
Ranch Buttermilk Gourmet
Ranch Reduced Calorie

Toppings:
Almond
Cashew
Chocolate Flake
Culver's Hot Fudge
M & M's Minis
Peanut Butter
Pecan Halves
Reese's® Peanut Butter Cups
Snickers® Candy Bar Pieces
Spanish Peanuts

Drinks: *(their iced and hot teas are listed as containing gluten)*
Culver's® Root Beer
Chocolate Milk Low Fat
Diet Pepsi®
Dr. Pepper®
Milk – 2%
Mocha N'iced Coffee™
Mountain Dew®
Pepsi®
Sierra Mist
Tropicana Fruit Punch®
Tropicana Pink Lemonade
Vanilla N'iced Coffee™
Wild Cherry Pepsi®

Shakes and Floats:
Culver's Root Beer Float
Vanilla Shake

Seasonal:
Pumpkin Shake

Special Treats:
Cooler
Lemon Ice
Lemon Ice Smoothie

Concrete Mixers:
Vanilla Concrete Mixer
Pumpkin Pecan Concrete Mixer

Disclaimer: We do not guarantee, nor do these restaurants guarantee that any menu item will be 100% gluten-free. These restaurants & Business Graphics Group assume no liability for your use of this information. See full disclaimer on page 7.

Dairy Queen

We know dealing with gluten intolerance can be very difficult and Dairy Queen would like to help you enjoy your favorite Dairy Queen treats while still following a safe diet. We hope the following information will be of assistance to you. If you are looking for something other than the products listed, please check out our nutrition calculator at the link below: http://dairyqueen.com/us-en/eats-and-treats/nutrition-calculator/ Our nutrition calculator offers nutrition, ingredients, and allergen information for all approved products within the Dairy Queen system. The nutrition calculator is continually updated with the newest information on products and promotions; as we strive to provide the most accurate, up-to-date information.

Gluten Free Choices: DQ vanilla and chocolate soft serve are gluten-free, in addition to our Arctic RushT slush. Additionally the following toppings are gluten-free: Chocolate, Hot Fudge, Marshmallow, Butterscotch, Strawberry. You may also want to try our one of our vanilla, mocha, or caramel MooLattes® *without whipped topping.*

Additionally, our supplier of manufactured novelties informs us that the following items are also gluten-free: DQ® Fudge Bar, DQ® Vanilla Orange Bar, Dilly® Bar and Buster® Bar (look for this in a sealed plastic wrap to ensure it is a manufactured Dilly Bar or Buster® Bar), Starkiss Bars

Gluten-free Blizzards: Reese's® Peanut Butter Cup Blizzard, Butterfinger® Blizzard, Heath® Blizzard, M&M® Blizzard, Banana Split Blizzard, Hawaiian Blizzard, Tropical Blizzard, Strawberry Blizzard

From our Brazier food line, I would recommend trying our Homestyle® and GrillBurgers, or our hot dogs, *all prepared without a bun.*

Please know many of our Blizzard candies and toppings contain wheat, rye, oats, and/or barley and would not be safe for a customer with gluten intolerance. As the Blizzard machine is used for all flavors, cross-contact may occur on any flavor Blizzard. So for your safety, we recommend notifying the Dairy Queen staff of your allergy or intolerance and requesting they thoroughly clean the Blizzard machine before blending your Blizzard to reduce the risk of cross-contact.

Certain Dairy Queen restaurants use a soft serve mix that varies from the mix used by restaurants in the rest of the country and on which this information is based. Please know some Dairy Queen restaurants also sell food that is not the licensed Brazier line of food products. This information on food products applies only to the Brazier products served by authorized Brazier restaurants. Please check all of this information regarding food and treats with your local restaurant. Please note that as Dairy Queen stores and restaurants are very busy and there is always a chance of cross contact of gluten in any DQ product. To reduce the risk, please mention the nature of your allergy to the DQ crew member before placing your order.

Disclaimer: We do not guarantee, nor do these restaurants guarantee that any menu item will be 100% gluten-free. These restaurants & Business Graphics Group assume no liability for your use of this information. See full disclaimer on page 7.

Dave and Buster's

PRIOR TO PLACING YOUR ORDER, PLEASE ALERT YOUR SERVER TO YOUR FOOD ALLERGY OR SPECIAL DIETARY NEEDS. We have prepared this list of suggested menu items based on the advice of our QA & Food Safety Manager/Nutritionist along with the most current information from our food suppliers and their stated absence of wheat/gluten protein within these items. Please be aware that during normal kitchen operations involving shared cooking equipment and preparation areas, which may or may not include common fryer oil, the possibility exists for cross contact, therefore, food items (including garnishes may come in contact with wheat/gluten proteins. Additionally, fried food items could absorb wheat/gluten proteins during the cooking process. Therefore, we recommend that individuals with these allergies and intolerances avoid ALL fried foods & garnishes. Due to these circumstances, we are unable to guarantee that any menu entrée below can be COMPLETELY free of wheat/gluten protein. *As an added precaution, please ask to be seated away from the kitchen to avoid potentially irritating aromas

Suggested Menu Options for Wheat/Gluten Allergies

Soups:
Beef Broth
Chicken Broth

Salads : (without Dressing & Tortilla Strips)
Sweet Apple Pecan Salad (Shrimp or Chicken)
Honey Mustard Spinach Salad
House Salad
Grilled Steak Salad (*no Frazzled Onions*)

Salad Dressings:
Oil & Vinegar

Chicken & Seafood: *(without Sides)*
Plain Grilled Chicken
Lacy's Chicken
Baked or Grilled Salmon

Sides:
Sauteed Green Beans
Mixed Vegetable Medley
Edamame

Buster's Burgers: *(without Fries or Bun)*
Bar Burger
Buster's Cheeseburger
Dave's Double Cheeseburgers
Monterey Burger

Grilled Steaks: *(without Sides & No Frazzled Onions)*
NY Strip
Sirloin Steak
Chargrilled NY Strip
Chargrilled Sirloin Steak

Sauces & Extras:
Guacamole
Pico de Gallo
Salsa
Sour Cream

Kids:
Kids Burger *(no Bun, no fries)*
Grilled Chicken

Disclaimer: We do not guarantee, nor do these restaurants guarantee that any menu item will be 100% gluten-free. These restaurants & Business Graphics Group assume no liability for your use of this information. See full disclaimer on page 7.

Dave and Buster's Continued:

At Dave & Buster's, the health and safety of our guests is always a top priority. As part of our on-going commitment to our guests with allergen concerns, we try to provide the most current information available from our suppliers on the eight most common allergens, not to exclude those with Wheat/Gluten Protein Intolerance. For more information about food allergies, feel free to contact our QA & Food Safety Mgr/Nutritionist, kevin_willis@daveandbusters.com or the Food Allergy Network Anaphylaxis Network: www.foodallergy.org

---

Disclaimer: We do not guarantee, nor do these restaurants guarantee that any menu item will be 100% gluten-free. These restaurants & Business Graphics Group assume no liability for your use of this information. See full disclaimer on page 7.

Denny's

Menu Items for Gluten Intolerance *This Information Has Been Prepared For Persons Who Must Restrict Gluten In Their Diets. These are food items that according to manufactures ingredient listing provided to Denny's and found to be free of gluten and gliaden, and products containing them such as soy sauce, unspecified food starches and vegetable proteins.*

Entree/Salads:
Eggs/Omelets
Side Garden Salad(*Request no croutons/dressing*)
Sliced/Shaved Ham
2 Egg & more breakfast w/hash browns (*no bread*)
Steak
Grilled Tilapia w/lemon butter sauce (*no rice pilaf*)
Beef Patty
Ultimate Omelette w/hash browns (*no bread*)
Bacon
Bacon Cheddar Burger patty/ w side of grapes (*no bun*)

Cereals:
Oatmeal [*for those who feel they can tolerate – these are not "gluten-free" oats*]
Grits
These items are produced & packaged in a plant that also produce and package wheat products

Sides/ Sauces:
Applesauce
Cottage Cheese
Fresh Fruit
Tomato Slices
Mashed Potatoes/Cheese
Green Beans
Olives
Salsa
High Div'n Veggies(*no breadsticks/ or dip*)
Garden Salad (*w/o croutons and dressing*)
Hashed Browns
Tartar Sauce
Corn
Pinto Beans (regional item)
Black-eyed Peas
Red Grapes
Pico de Gallo
Sliced Cucumbers
Celery Sticks
Jump-shot Jello
Seasonal Fruit
Lemon Butter Sauce
Baby Carrots (raw)

Disclaimer: We do not guarantee, nor do these restaurants guarantee that any menu item will be 100% gluten-free. These restaurants & Business Graphics Group assume no liability for your use of this information. See full disclaimer on page 7.

Page | **54**

Denny's Continued:

Vanilla Yogurt
*Regular French Fries
*Fried Corn Tortilla (used in Nachos)
*Please verify that dedicated fryers are used for french fries & tortillas before you order.

Miscellaneous:
American Processed Cheese
Butter
Cherry Flavoring
Swiss Processed Cheese
Cheese
Reduced Cal. French Dressing
Cheddar Cheese
Banana
Cottage Cheese/purchased locally check label
Cream Cheese
Strawberries
Liquid &Whipped Margarine
Maraschino Cherries
Honey
Lemon wedges
Lime wedges
Pancake/Waffle Syrup
Red wine Vinegar
Strawberry, Grape, Mixed Fruit Jelly

Beverages:
Milk- all except buttermilk, Grapefruit Juice. Lemonade, Coke, Orange Juice, Tomato Juice, Tea& Tea Chillers, Root Beer, Raspberry Tea, Hot Chocolate, Sprite, Diet Coke, Flavored Coffees, Dr. Pepper, Fusion Favorites, Coffee

This guidance sheet is developed using commonly recognized foods and food components. In addition to the terms listed at the top of the guidance sheet please inquire about and inspect labels using any terms provided by your allergist or doctor, and speak with your server/manager regarding issues of cross-contamination. Depending on your order, request that they wash the grill or fry your potatoes, or meat in an omelet pan to avoid cross contamination. ***Always*** *inform your server or speak to the manager regarding specific needs prior to placing your order. This listing is based on information provided by product vendors and specifications, and may not be all inclusive. Please be aware that vendors and product formulations may change. Also some locations may use different vendors or local vendors. If you are concerned about an ingredient ask store personnel for information before you order! If necessary, product labels are available. This list is updated periodically, for an update or further questions please call the nutrition coordinator at (864) 597-7396. Revised May 2010*

Disclaimer: We do not guarantee, nor do these restaurants guarantee that any menu item will be 100% gluten-free. These restaurants & Business Graphics Group assume no liability for your use of this information. See full disclaimer on page 7.

Dunkin Donuts (beverage info)

The following information about gluten-free menu items has been obtained either from the restaurant's website or through direct contact with guest services via email or phone.

Except for our smoothies, all of our beverages are gluten free.

Disclaimer: We do not guarantee, nor do these restaurants guarantee that any menu item will be 100% gluten-free. These restaurants & Business Graphics Group assume no liability for your use of this information. See full disclaimer on page 7.

Eat 'n Park

The following information about gluten-free menu items has been obtained either from the restaurant's website or through direct contact with guest services via email or phone.

For those of our guests who cannot eat food with gluten (wheat, rye, and barley products), we have a wide variety of menu items that can meet your special dietary needs.

**Please note: To avoid cross-contact with gluten ingredients, please let your server know that you are requesting a gluten-free item.

Our fried items are not gluten-free - our fryers are used to fry breaded items. While we make every effort to ensure our celiac-friendly items do not come into contact with other ingredients, we cannot guarantee that our cooking surfaces are completely gluten-free.

New Gluten Free Bun: Our celiac-friendly rice/tapioca-based bun is similar to an Italian style roll, and can be substituted in place of the bread/bun on any of our sandwiches, breakfast sandwiches, or burgers.

Ingredients: Filtered water, rice flour, corn starch, tapioca starch, eggs, expeller pressed canola oil, potato starch, sugar. Contains less than 2% of the following: yeast, protein replacer [potato starch, tapioca flour, leavening (calcium lactate), calcium carbonate, citric acid, carbohydrate gum], salt, xanthan gum, organic apple cider vinegar.

Breakfast:
Fresh Fruit Cup
Strawberries (in season)
Home fries
Sausage
Bacon
Ham
Canadian Bacon
Maple Syrup

Cheese Omelette: *no toast*
Eat'n Smart Smile: *no toast*
Eggs Benedict: *no English muffin*
Eggs Breakfast: *no toast*
Ham and Cheese Omelette: no *toast*
Meat Lover's Omelette: *without toast*
Original Breakfast Smile: *no toast*
Super Omelette Smile: *without toast*
T-Bone Steak & Eggs Smile: *no toast*
Veggie Omelette: *without toast*
Western Omelette: *without toast*

Salad Dressings:
All dressings served at Eat'n Park are gluten-free
Salads:
Chicken Fajita Salad: *without tortilla bowl*
Grilled Chicken Portabella Salad: *without croutons*
Grilled Chicken Salad: *without French fries*

Burgers:
Black Angus American Grill Burger: *without Texas toast*
Black Angus BBQ Bacon and Cheddar Burger: *without the bun*
Black Angus Mushroom & Onion Burger: *without the bun*
Black Angus Superburger: *without the bun*
Classic Black Angus Burger: *without Kaiser roll*

Disclaimer: We do not guarantee, nor do these restaurants guarantee that any menu item will be 100% gluten-free. These restaurants & Business Graphics Group assume no liability for your use of this information. See full disclaimer on page 7.

Eat 'n Park Continued:

Celiac-Friendly Sides:
Homemade Chili
Garden Salad (*no croutons*)
Mashed Potatoes (*no gravy*)
Seasonal Vegetables
Fresh Broccoli
Cottage Cheese
Apple Sauce
Fresh Fruit Cup (in season)
Baked Potato

Dinners:
Baked Cod: *without bread crumbs and dinner rolls*
Beef Liver & Onions: *without dinner rolls*
Chargrilled Chicken: *without dinner rolls*
Chargrilled Sockeye Salmon: *without dinner rolls*
Chicken Stir-fry: *without garden rice*
Eat'n Smart Cod Floridian: *without seasoning and without dinner rolls*
Ground Sirloin Steak: *without onion rings*
T-Bone Steak

Disclaimer: We do not guarantee, nor do these restaurants guarantee that any menu item will be 100% gluten-free. These restaurants & Business Graphics Group assume no liability for your use of this information. See full disclaimer on page 7.

El Pollo Loco

The following information about gluten-free menu items has been obtained either from the restaurant's website or through direct contact with guest services via email or phone.

Pinto Beans
Refried beans
Cotija cheese
Mixed Vegetables
Corn tortillas (Does contain corn gluten)

Flame grilled Mexican chicken - No wheat gluten, however it *IS chopped on the same chopping board as other chicken items that do contain wheat gluten.*

Avocado Salsa does **not** contain wheat, barley or rye gluten.

The Flan served at El Pollo Loco does not contain gluten at this time.

The Buffaloco Wings served at El Pollo Loco do not contain gluten at this time

BBQ Chicken Flavor Event does not contain gluten. *The product however is prepared on the same cutting board and uses common utensils as other chicken products that may contain gluten. Depending on your level of sensitivity, this may or may not be a consideration.*

Disclaimer: We do not guarantee, nor do these restaurants guarantee that any menu item will be 100% gluten-free. These restaurants & Business Graphics Group assume no liability for your use of this information. See full disclaimer on page 7.

Firehouse Subs

The following information about gluten-free menu items has been obtained either from the restaurant's website or through direct contact with guest services via email or phone.

Salads/Soups/Meats/Sides:
Chili
Chief's Salad w/ Ham
Chief's Salad w/ Turkey
Ham
Turkey
Pastrami
Chicken Breast (Sliced)
Roast Beef
Corned Beef
Steak
Pepperoni
Salami
Bacon
Brisket
Mushrooms
Au jus onions and peppers
Pickles
Marinara sauce
Chips – see packaging

Dressings:
Mayo
Honey Mustard
Italian Dressing
Thousand Island Dressing
Balsamic Dressing
Raspberry Vinaigrette
Ranch Dressing
Fat Free Ranch Dressing
Mustard (brown and yellow)
Capt. Sorensen Sauce
Fresh lettuce, tomato, onions
Black olives
Banana peppers
Jalapeno peppers
Cheese (all varieties)

Disclaimer: We do not guarantee, nor do these restaurants guarantee that any menu item will be 100% gluten-free. These restaurants & Business Graphics Group assume no liability for your use of this information. See full disclaimer on page 7.

First Watch

Gluten Free Diet Information: The following includes a comprehensive list of menu items at First Watch that are Gluten-Free. However, due to occasional product substitutions or potential for changes in product ingredients without the knowledge of First Watch, Gluten intolerant guests are urged to use tremendous care in choosing from our menu. First Watch provides this menu information as a service to our customers. First Watch assumes no responsibility for its use and any resulting liability or consequential damages is denied. A Registered Dietitian prepared this information (which has not been verified by First Watch Restaurants). Patrons are encouraged to consider this information in light of their individual requirements and needs.

Egg-Cetera: (*order without bread/sauce*)
Breakfast Scramble – *No croissant, No Hollandaise sauce*
Bubba's Benny - *No biscuits, No sausage gravy, No English Muffin*
Caps Mushroom – *No English muffin*
Chickichanga – *No flour tortilla, No Vera Cruz sauce*
Avocado Skillet - *No English muffin*
Ham Skillet - *No English muffin*
Onion Skillet - *No English muffin*
Veggie Skillet - *No English muffin*
Eggs Benedict Florentine - *No English muffin, No Hollandaise sauce*
Eggs Benedict Ham - *No English muffin, No Hollandaise sauce*
Eggs Benedict Turkey - *No English muffin, No Hollandaise sauce*
Joaquin Yahoo - *No English muffin*
Sonoran Fritatta - *No English muffin*
Burrito Vera Cruz - *No flour tortilla, No Vera Cruz sauce*

Eggs and Omelettes: (*no English muffin*)
Acapulco Express - *No English muffin*
Bacado – *No English muffin*
Ham / Bacon / Sausage / and Cheese Omelette– *No English muffin*
Greek Fetish - *No English muffin*
Killer Cajun – *No English muffin, No Santa Fe dressing*
Mushroom Omelette – *No English muffin*
The Works – *No English muffin*
Traditional- *No English muffin*

Sandwiches: (*order without bread/roll/bun*)
All meats are gluten free. *All breads, rolls, buns, croissants and muffins and wraps at First Watch contain Gluten.*
*Note - if you bring in your own Gluten Free bread, we will serve you a breadless sandwich so you can "build your own"; please do not attempt to send your bread to the kitchen as this could result in cross-contamination.
Al B. Core - *No bread*
BCB Burger - *No Kaiser roll or bread*
Beefeater - *No bread*
BLTE - *No bread*
Chicken Salad Melt - *No bread*
Turkey Burger - *No dressing, No bread*
Monterey Club - *No croissant*
Not Guilty Your Honor - *No Flatbread*
Rueben - *No bread*
Grill Turkey - *No bread, No Ranch Dressing*
San Diego Chicken - *No wheat bun*

Wraps: (*order without wrap*)
Going Cold Turkey- *No Tortilla, No Ranch Dressing*
Black and Blue- *No Tortilla, No horseradish sauce*
Green Hamlet Wrap– *No tortilla, No Honey Dijon dressing*
Heard of Buffalo Chicken - *No tortilla, No Ranch dressing*

Disclaimer: We do not guarantee, nor do these restaurants guarantee that any menu item will be 100% gluten-free. These restaurants & Business Graphics Group assume no liability for your use of this information. See full disclaimer on page 7.

First Watch Continued:

Veggie Omelette - *No English muffin*
Far West- *No English muffin*

Side List / Extras:
Gluten Free- Ham / Bacon / Sausage / Turkey Sausage/ Turkey Patty/ Potatoes/ Salad Marinade/ Fruit cup/ Salsa

Health Department:
Fruit Bowl is Gluten Free
Siesta Key Cocktail - *no granola, no muffin*
Power Wrap- *no tortilla wrap*
Tri-Athlete - *no muffin*
Lean Machine- *no muffin*
Healthy Turkey Omelette- *No English muffin*

Salad Bowl: **note: salad dressings that are available at First Watch vary according to location. In general, many pre-made dressings contain trace amounts of gluten; and therefore, caution should be used in choosing these products.*
Gluten Free dressings: House Dressing (Poppy Seed Vinaigrette), Greek, Sweet and Sour, and oil and vinegar (wine, cider or rice.)

Pecan Dijon Salad- *No pita, No Honey Dijon dressing*
Fruity Chicken Salad - *No pita*
Cobb Salad - *No pita*
Santa Fe Salad - *No dressing, No croutons, No pita*

Kids Menu:
Bacon and Egg – *without toast*
Hot Dog – *without bun or croissant*

Special note: The list above DOES NOT include several of our products that contain distilled vinegar. Several older publications list distilled vinegar as a product for the gluten intolerant to avoid while most new information suggests distilled vinegar is safe to consume. If you are concerned about this particular product, then you should avoid ALL dressings, mayonnaise, mustard, ketchup, chicken salad, tuna salad, and chorizo sausage, horseradish.

Disclaimer: We do not guarantee, nor do these restaurants guarantee that any menu item will be 100% gluten-free. These restaurants & Business Graphics Group assume no liability for your use of this information. See full disclaimer on page 7.

Five Guys Burgers and Fries

The following information about gluten-free menu items has been obtained either from the restaurant's website or through direct contact with guest services via email or phone.

The buns contain gluten, but the rest of the menu does not, including the fries.

Burgers: (*order without the bun*)
Hamburger
Cheeseburger
Bacon burger
Bacon cheeseburger
Little hamburger
Little cheeseburger
Little bacon burger
Little bacon cheeseburger

Dogs: (*order without the bun*)
Kosher style hot dog
Cheese *or* bacon dog
Bacon cheese dog

Fries:
Five guys style
Cajun

Toppings:
Mayo
Relish
Onions
Lettuce
Pickles
Tomatoes
Grilled Onions
Grilled Mushrooms
Ketchup
Mustard
Jalapeno Peppers
Green Peppers
A-1 Sauce
Bar-B-Q Sauce
Hot Sauce

Disclaimer: We do not guarantee, nor do these restaurants guarantee that any menu item will be 100% gluten-free. These restaurants & Business Graphics Group assume no liability for your use of this information. See full disclaimer on page 7.

Fleming's Prime Steakhouse & Wine Bar

The following information about gluten-free menu items has been obtained either from the restaurant's website or through direct contact with guest services via email or phone.

Gluten-Free Menu: *The recipes for the following menu items are gluten-free or can be ordered with the suggested changes to be gluten-free. The kitchen at Fleming's is not gluten-free. Tell your server you are ordering gluten-free.*

Appetizers:
Tenderloin Carpaccio - *Order without croutons.*
Wicked Cajun Barbecue Shrimp - *Order without croutons.*
Cheese Plate - *Order without bread.*
Shrimp Cocktail - *Order as is.*
Chilled Seafood - *Do not use creamy mustard sauce.*
Seared Ahi Tuna - *Order without Spicy Mustard*. Substitute with Caper Creole Mustard.

Soups:
The following soups are gluten-free:
Butternut Squash
Cream of Broccoli
Cream of Asparagus
Lobster Bisque

Salads: *Order all salads without croutons.*
All salad dressings are gluten-free except the Red Onion Balsamic.

Dinner Sides:
Acceptable sides:
Baked Potato
Fleming's Potatoes
Mashed Potatoes - Parmesan-peppercorn, blue cheese compound butters or roasted garlic.
Sautéed Spinach
Sautéed Mushrooms
Grilled Asparagus
Sugar Snap Peas - *Order without Soy Chili Glaze.*
Note: *Double Cut Shoestring Potatoes are not recommended due to possible cross-contamination in the fryer.*

Dinner Entrées with Meat:
All entrées can be ordered.
NY Strip
Tuscan Veal Chop - *Order grilled or sautéed without breading using olive oil.* Tomato, Basil, Olive Oil topping is acceptable.
Steak Sandwich - *order without the bread and ask that the vegetables be prepared without the Soy Chili Glaze.*

Lunch Entrées with Meat:
Prime Chopped Sirloin Steak
Italian Chicken Breast - *Order without panko crumbs and with acceptable side*

Seafood:
Barbeque Scottish Salmon Fillet - *Order with acceptable side and without Barbeque glaze*
Seared Scallops - *Order without the pastry.*
Lobster En Fuego - *Order with extra seared lemon instead of Lobster En Fuego Sauce and no croutons*
Australian Lobster - Order as is
Alaskan King Crab - Order as is
Tuna Mignon - Order as is

Sandwiches: (Lunch Only)
Prime Sirloin Burger - *without the Kaiser Roll*
Shaved Rosemary Chicken - *without the Kaiser Roll*
Steak Sandwich - *order without the Sourdough Roll and ask that the vegetables be prepared without the Soy Chili Glaze*
French Dip - *without bread*

Disclaimer: We do not guarantee, nor do these restaurants guarantee that any menu item will be 100% gluten-free. These restaurants & Business Graphics Group assume no liability for your use of this information. See full disclaimer on page 7.

Fleming's Continued:

Lunch Sides:
Cole Slaw
Cracked Potatoes
Sugar Snap Peas - *Order without Soy Chili Glaze.*

Desserts:
Crème Brulée
Mixed berries with whipped cream and/or vanilla ice cream
Vanilla ice cream with choice of the following sauces:
Raspberry Sauce
Fudge Sauce

Disclaimer: We do not guarantee, nor do these restaurants guarantee that any menu item will be 100% gluten-free. These restaurants & Business Graphics Group assume no liability for your use of this information. See full disclaimer on page 7.

Friendly's

Here is a list of menu items that do not contain wheat, rye or barley (oats are not included on this list).

Ice Cream Flavors:
- Vanilla
- Strawberry
- Chocolate
- Coffee
- Forbidden Chocolate®
- Vienna Mocha Chunk®
- Mint Chocolate Chip
- Purely Pistachio®
- Chocolate Chip
- Black Raspberry
- Butter Pecan
- Butter Crunch
- Chocolate Almond Chip
- Maple Walnut
- No Sugar Added Vanilla
- Vanilla Fat-Free Yogurt
- Raspberry Fat-Free Swirl Yogurt
- Orange Sherbet
- Watermelon Sherbet
- Soft Serve (Vanilla, Chocolate or Twist)
- Peanut Butter Cup (Limited Time Only)

Toppings:
- Hot Fudge
- Strawberry
- Marshmallow
- Chocolate Syrup
- Peanut Butter
- Sprinkles (Chocolate or Rainbow)
- Cherry
- Swiss Chocolate
- Caramel
- No Sugar Added Fudge
- Whipped Topping
- Almonds
- Walnuts
- Banana
- Reese's® Pieces™
- Reese's® Peanut Butter Cups™
- Crushed Health® Bar (with Almonds)
- Gummy Bears
- M&M's®
- Butterfinger® Pieces

Fountain Beverages:
- Double Thick Milk Shakes (Vanilla, Chocolate, Strawberry or Coffee)
- Fribble® (Vanilla, Chocolate, Strawberry or Butterfinger®)
- Barq's® Float
- Watermelon or Orange Slammer™

Desserts:
- Kids Hot Fudge
- Monster Mash Sundae
- Jim Dandy
- Peanut Butter Cup Sundae
- Ultimate Peanut Butter Cup Sundae
- Butterfinger® Sundae
- Fruit and Sherbet Sundae
- Reese's® Pieces™ Sundae
- Health® Bar Friend-Z®
- M&M's® Friend-Z®
- Reese's® Peanut Butter Cup™ Friend-Z®
- Strawberry Banana Friend-Z®
- Butterfinger Friend-z®
- Peanut Butter Cup Friend-Z®
- Royal Banana Split

Entrées: Sirloin Steak Tips or Cheddar Jack Chicken

Sides:
- Mashed Potatoes
- Mixed Vegetables with Margarine
- Whole Kernel Corn with Margarine
- Rice
- Cole Slaw
- Applesauce
- Mandarin Oranges
- Bacon
- Sausage Link
- Hickory-Smoked Ham
- Broccoli with Margarine

Disclaimer: We do not guarantee, nor do these restaurants guarantee that any menu item will be 100% gluten-free. These restaurants & Business Graphics Group assume no liability for your use of this information. See full disclaimer on page 7.

Friendly's Continued:

Dressings and Condiments:

Bleu Cheese Dressing	A-1 Steak Sauce	Relish
Buttermilk Ranch	Cocktail Sauce	Salsa
Caesar Dressing	Mustard (Spicy Brown	Tartar Sauce
Honey Mustard	and Yellow)	Worcestershire Sauce
Italian Fat-Free	Ketchup	Pickle Chips
Italian Style	Marinara Sauce	Roasted Pepper Garlic
Thousand Island		Sauce

Friendly's works hard to provide current and accurate information on ingredients in our menu items that may be potential food allergens for some customers. We prepared this brochure to provide you important information to help you make careful choices when dining in our restaurant. We examined the ingredients in each of our standard recipes in order to list the eight most common food allergens identified by the U.S. Food and Drug Administration. However, this brochure is not intended to address other, less common allergens, and doesn't include regional products, or local specials. Our suppliers or ingredients may change without notice, and any requested additions or substitutions to menu items could also change the potential allergen content. In addition, common restaurant cooking equipment, such as grills and fryers, may create a risk of allergen residue from food cross-contact. We exercise great care to minimize this risk, but it cannot be eliminated entirely. If you have a question about a menu item, ingredients or preparation, please ask your server. We recommend that you consult your medical professional with any concerns you have about food allergies and/or food sensitivities. If you would like further information regarding special sensitivities or dietary concerns, please contact us at Friendly Ice Cream Corp., 1855 Boston Road, Wilbraham, MA 01095, (800) 966-9970 or visit us at www.friendlys.com. VALID AS OF JUNE 16, 2008.

Disclaimer: We do not guarantee, nor do these restaurants guarantee that any menu item will be 100% gluten-free. These restaurants & Business Graphics Group assume no liability for your use of this information. See full disclaimer on page 7.

Golden Corral

The following information about gluten-free menu items has been obtained either from the restaurant's website or through direct contact with guest services via email or phone.

Please refer to the below listing of products that are gluten free in our restaurants. This list is currently being updated, so if there are items not listed, please let me know and I can check those for you. Also, due to our restaurants containing all 'Big 8' allergens in-house, we cannot guarantee cross contamination in our stores. This is especially true, since customers serve themselves. Thanks for choosing Golden Corral.

Proteins:
Carved Turkey
Sausage (Italian Roped and Cajun)
Grilled Pork Chops
Turkey Strips, Cold
Ham Strips, Cold
Sirloin
Beef Brisket
Ham, Pitt
BBQ Pork Ribs
Flame Broiled Glazed Pork Ribs
Pork Loin Roast
Salmon, Whole Carved
BBQ Chicken (Leg Quarter)
BBQ Pork
Rotisserie Chicken (Breast and Wing)
Pulled Chicken (Salad Bar)

Vegetables/Side Dishes:
Sugar Snap Peas
Key West Blend
Creamed Spinach
Creamed Corn
Mashed Potatoes
Broccoli
Cauliflower
Baked Potato
Baked Sweet Potato (*but Sweet Potato Casserole contains Gluten*)
Wild Rice (*but Rice Pilaf contains Gluten*)

Promotions:
Oceans of Shrimp
Baked Fish with Shrimp and Lemon Herb Sauce
Shrimp Scampi

Miscellaneous:
Solid Margarine
BBQ Sauce
Cajun Mayo
Oil & Vinegar
Caesar Dressing
Mayonnaise
Cole Slaw
Ranch Dressing
Dijon Honey Mustard
French Dressing
Fat Free French Dressing
Fat Free Ranch Dressing
Blue Cheese Dressing

Breakfast:
Scrambled Eggs
Liquid Eggs
Whole Eggs
Corned Beef Hash
Bacon
Breakfast Links
Split Smoked Sausage
Breakfast Sausage Patties
Shredded Hash Browns
Orange Juice
Apple Juice
Orange Guava juice

Disclaimer: We do not guarantee, nor do these restaurants guarantee that any menu item will be 100% gluten-free. These restaurants & Business Graphics Group assume no liability for your use of this information. See full disclaimer on page 7.

Golden Corral Continued:

Applewood Grill:
Spinach Applewood Bacon Salad

Great American Seafood Tour:
Salmon Lemonata
Tilapia Florentine
Grilled Lemon Pepper Tilapia

Desserts:
Sugar Free Jell-O
Sugar Free Pudding
Chocolate Icing
Whipped On Top
Vanilla Soft Serve
Chocolate Soft Serve
Sherbets (Orange)
Candy Corn
Gummie Bears
Jelly Beans
Orange Slices

Disclaimer: We do not guarantee, nor do these restaurants guarantee that any menu item will be 100% gluten-free. These restaurants & Business Graphics Group assume no liability for your use of this information. See full disclaimer on page 7.

Hardee's

The following information about gluten-free menu items has been obtained either from the restaurant's website or through direct contact with guest services via email or phone.

List of Wheat-Free Menu Items (gluten is not listed on their allergen chart):

- Bacon
- Bacon Bits
- Beef Frank or Hot Dog (*no buns/bread*)
- Beef Patty
- Butter Packet
- Buttermilk
- Buttermilk Ranch Dressing
- American Cheese
- Cheddar Cheese, shredded
- Swiss Cheese
- Chili
- Coffee
- Cole Slaw
- Coffee Creamer
- Half and Half
- Eggs, Scrambled or Folded
- French Fries (natural Cut) – *ask if they are fried in a dedicated fryer*
- Grits
- Country Ham
- Diced Ham
- Sliced Ham
- Hot Chocolate
- Italian Dressing, Low Fat
- Ketchup
- Lettuce, Iceburg
- Little Thickburger Patty
- Liquid Margarine
- Mayonnaise
- Mustard Packet
- Onions: Red and Yellow
- Pancake Syrup
- Pickle Chips: Bread and Butter and Dill
- Mashed Potatoes
- Roast Beef
- Salsa Packet
- BBQ Sauce
- Horseradish Sauce
- Honey Mustard Sauce
- Mushroom Sauce
- House Ranch Sauce
- Hot n Sour Sauce
- Texas Pete's Hot Sauce
- Sausage Patty
- Tarter Sauce
- Tomato

Chocolate Ice Cream, Mint Chocolate Chip Ice Cream, Peach Ice Cream, Strawberry Ice Cream, Vanilla Ice Cream, Vanilla, Extra Creamy Ice Cream and Whipped Topping

Milkshake Syrups: Chocolate, Strawberry, Vanilla

Disclaimer: We do not guarantee, nor do these restaurants guarantee that any menu item will be 100% gluten-free. These restaurants & Business Graphics Group assume no liability for your use of this information. See full disclaimer on page 7.

In-N-Out Burger

The following information about gluten-free menu items has been obtained either from the restaurant's website or through direct contact with guest services via email or phone.

All of their foods are gluten-free except the buns, so you can order any burger "Protein Style" and they will replace the bun with Lettuce.

Hamburger Protein Style
Cheeseburger Protein Style
Double Double Protein Style
French Fries
Chocolate Shake
Vanilla Shake
Strawberry Shake

Disclaimer: We do not guarantee, nor do these restaurants guarantee that any menu item will be 100% gluten-free. These restaurants & Business Graphics Group assume no liability for your use of this information. See full disclaimer on page 7.

Islands Restaurant

The following information about gluten-free menu items has been obtained either from the restaurant's website or through direct contact with guest services via email or phone.

Islands cannot guarantee that any menu item will be prepared <u>completely</u> free of the allergen in question. Islands relied on our suppliers' statements of ingredients in deciding which products did not contain certain allergens. Suppliers may change the ingredients in their products or the way they prepare their products, so please check this list to make sure that the menu item still meets your dietary requirements. From time to time, we may substitute products due to inventory shortages. We cannot be certain that the substitute products will be free of the allergen you wish to avoid. As we cook, prepare, and serve your meal, the listed menu item may come in contact with the allergen you wish to avoid. For example, from time to time, we may cook products using shared cooking oil, or cook the listed menu option on the same grill as a menu item that contains the allergen you want to avoid.

The following items are gluten free:

Grilled Veggie Tacos w/corn tortillas
Grilled Chicken Tacos w/onion, peppers and corn tortillas (without ranchero beans)
Cabo Loco Tacos w/corn tortillas (without ranchero beans)
Kaanapali Kobb Salad without focaccia bread

Disclaimer: We do not guarantee, nor do these restaurants guarantee that any menu item will be 100% gluten-free. These restaurants & Business Graphics Group assume no liability for your use of this information. See full disclaimer on page 7.

Jamba Juice

The following information about gluten-free menu items has been obtained either from the restaurant's website or through direct contact with guest services via email or phone.

Allergen/Cross-contamination statement: Because many of our products are freshly made, trace amounts of allergens (like peanuts may be present in all products).

All smoothies are non-gluten *except for Pomegranate Heart Happy*.
All Boosts and Super Boosts are non-gluten (*except for Daily Vitamin, Energy and Heart Happy*).

- Probioitic Boost
- Coffee Craze
- Super Yumberry
- Berry Yumberry
- Chill-icious Chai
- Classic Hot Chocolate with Soy Milk
- Classic Hot Chocolate with 2% Milk
- Classic Hot Chocolate with Nonfat Milk
- Organic Detox Infusion
- Organic African Nectar
- Organic Spring Jasmine
- Organic Green Dragon
- Organic Earl Grey
- Organic Breakfast
- Heavenly Green Tea Latte with Soy Milk
- Heavenly Green Tea Latte with 2% Milk
- Heavenly Green Tea Latte with Nonfat Milk
- Perfectly Chocolate Chai Tea Latte with Soy Milk
- Perfectly Chocolate Chai Tea Latte with 2% Milk
- Perfectly Chocolate Chai Tea Latte with Nonfat Milk
- Original Spiced Chai Tea Latte with Soy Milk
- Original Spiced Chai Tea Latte with 2% Milk
- Original Spiced Chai Tea Latte with Nonfat Milk
- Five Fruit Frenzy
- Pomegranate Pick Me Up
- 3G Charger Super Boost
- Flax & Fiber Super Boost
- Matcha Energy Shot Soy Milk
- Matcha Energy Shot Orange Juice
- Protein Berry Workout with Whey
- Calcium Boost
- Whey Protein Super Boost
- Antioxidant Power Super Boost
- Soy Protein Boost
- Immunity Boost
- Carrot Juice
- Orange Juice
- Orange Dream Machine
- Aloha Pineapple
- Caribbean Passion
- Mango-a-go-go
- Peach Pleasure
- Banana Berry
- Razzmatazz
- Strawberry Surf Rider
- Strawberries Wild
- Peanut Butter Moo'd
- Chocolate Moo'd
- Matcha Green Tea Blast
- Acai Super-Antioxidant
- Protein Berry Workout w/ Soy Protein
- Coldbuster
- Mango Mantra
- Strawberry Nirvana
- Mega Mango
- Strawberry Whirl
- Peach Perfection
- Pomegranate Paradise

Disclaimer: We do not guarantee, nor do these restaurants guarantee that any menu item will be 100% gluten-free. These restaurants & Business Graphics Group assume no liability for your use of this information. See full disclaimer on page 7.

Jersey Mike's Subs

The following information about gluten-free menu items has been obtained either from the restaurant's website or through direct contact with guest services via email or phone.

Meats:
#1 BLT in a Tub
#2 Jersey Shore Favorite in a Tub
#3 American Classic in a Tub
#4 in a Tub
#5 Super Sub in a Tub
#6 Roast Beef & Provolone in a Tub
#7 Turkey Breast & Provolone in a Tub
#8 Club Sub in a Tub with mayo
#9 Club Supreme in a Tub with mayo
#10 Albacore Tuna in a Tub
#11 in a Tub
#12 in a Tub
#13 Original Italian in a Tub
#14 Veggie in a Tub

Salads:
Tossed Salad (*no dressing*)
Chef Salad (*no dressing*)
Grilled Chicken Caesar Salad
Tuna Salad (*no dressing*)

Components:
American Cheese, Pasteurized
Parmesan Cheese, Grated
Pepper Jack Cheese
Provolone Cheese
Swiss Cheese
Banana Peppers
Blended Oil
Buffalo Sauce
Chipotle Mayonnaise
Dijon Honey Mustard
Dill Pickle
Green Peppers
Jalapeno Peppers
Lettuce
Mayonnaise
Onion
Red Wine Vinegar
Sauerkraut
Spaghetti Sauce
Tomato
Bacon
Chicken Breast, Grilled
Ham, Boiled
Ham, Capicolla
Ham Proscuittini Peppered
Pastrami
Pepperoni, Deli
Philly Chicken
Philly Steak
Roast Beef
Salami, hard
Sausage, Italian
Sausage Patty, Breakfast
Tuna Fish Salad
Turkey Breast, Oven Roasted

Salad Dressings:
Blue Cheese
Caesar
Chipotle Mayo
Golden Italian
Italian Fat Free
Ranch
Russian

Disclaimer: We do not guarantee, nor do these restaurants guarantee that any menu item will be 100% gluten-free. These restaurants & Business Graphics Group assume no liability for your use of this information. See full disclaimer on page 7.

Johnny Rockets

Johnny Rockets products feature ingredients which may contain wheat flour and/or gluten. If your condition is life threatening then it may be in your best interest to avoid our restaurant due to the possible, however extremely unlikely, event that residue from contraindicated products may come in contact with those considered "safe." We are in contact with the Celiac Disease Foundation as well as the Celiac Sprue Association in order to obtain more information.

List of Wheat-Free Menu Items (gluten is not listed on their allergen chart):

Almonds
American Cheese
Ancho Chipotle Sauce Bacon
Balsamic Vinaigarette Dressing
Bananas
Barq's® Root Beer
BBQ Sauce
Beef Steak
Black Pepper
Blue Cheese Dressing
Butterfinger® Pieces
Butter Flavored Seasoning
Cheddar Cheese
Cheddar Cheese (shredded)
Cherry Syrup
Chicken Breast
Chicken of the Sea Tuna
Cocoa Mix
Coffee - Decaf
Coffee - Regular
Coffee-flavored Shake Base
Coke®
Cream Cheese
Creamer - Half & Half
Creamy Ceasar Dressing
Diet Coke®
Dijon Mustard
Dijonnaise Sauce
Eggs - Fresh
Equal®
Fajita Blend 3/8" Strips
Fanta® Orange Soda
Grape Jelly
Gulden's® Mustard
Ham
Hamburger Patty
Hard Boiled Eggs
Hershey's® Chocolate Syrup
Italian (fat-free) Dressing
Ketchup
Ketchup - Packet
Lipton® Iced & Hot Tea
Lemonade
Lemons
Lettuce - Iceberg
Lettuce - Romaine
Mayonnaise
Mushrooms
Mustard
OJ
Onion Powder
Onions
Peanut Butter
Pepper Jack Cheese
Pepper Relish Sauce
Pibb® Xtra
Pickle
Pickle Relish
Pineapple Dessert Topping
Red Red® Sauce
"Rocket Fuel" Rocket Wing Sauce
Salt
Sanka
Sausage
Secret Seasoning
Slider Patties
Special Sauce
Sprite®
St. Louis Sauce
Strawberry Shake Base
Strawberry Topping
Sugar
Sweet'N Low®
Swiss Cheese
Tabasco Sauce
Thousand Island Dressing

Disclaimer: We do not guarantee, nor do these restaurants guarantee that any menu item will be 100% gluten-free. These restaurants & Business Graphics Group assume no liability for your use of this information. See full disclaimer on page 7.

Johnny Rocket's Continued:

Hi-C® Fruit Punch
Honey
Honey Mustard Dressing
Hot Fudge

Tomatoes
Turkey Patty
"Traditional" Rocket Wing Sauce
Vanilla Ice Cream
Vanilla Syrup
Whipped Cream
Whole Milk

Disclaimer: We do not guarantee, nor do these restaurants guarantee that any menu item will be 100% gluten-free. These restaurants & Business Graphics Group assume no liability for your use of this information. See full disclaimer on page 7.

Kentucky Fried Chicken

The following information about gluten-free menu items has been obtained either from the restaurant's website or through direct contact with guest services via email or phone.

Here's a list of the menu items that do not contain gluten (*none of their chicken is gluten-free*):

Salads:
Caesar side salad *without dressing and without croutons*
House side salad *without dressing*

Sides:
Green Beans
Seasoned Rice
Corn on the Cob
Potato Salad
Sweet Kernel Corn
KFC Mean Greens

Dressings, Sauces and Misc:
Heinz ® Buttermilk Ranch Dressing
Hidden Valley ® The Original Ranch ® Fat Free Dressing
Marzetti ® Light Italian Dressing
KFC ® Creamy Parmesan Caesar Dressing
Pre-Shredded Lettuce
Tomato Slices
Monterey Jack Cheese Slices
Honey BBQ Sandwich Sauce
Pepper Mayonnaise
Spicy Mayonnaise
Garlic Parmesan Dipping Sauce
Sweet and Sour Dipping Sauce
Honey Mustard Dipping Sauce
Creamy Ranch Dipping Sauce
BBQ Dipping Sauce
Jalapeno Peppers

Disclaimer: We do not guarantee, nor do these restaurants guarantee that any menu item will be 100% gluten-free. These restaurants & Business Graphics Group assume no liability for your use of this information. See full disclaimer on page 7.

Krystal

The following information about gluten-free menu items has been obtained either from the restaurant's website or through direct contact with guest services via email or phone.

Krystal nutrition information is from an independent lab, combined with representative values from Krystal food suppliers, USDA, and other established databases. This information is based on standard product formulations, averages or both. Variations may occur due to differences in suppliers, ingredient substitutions, recipe revisions, product assembly at the restaurant level, and/or season of the year. Some menu items may not be available at all restaurants. Test products, test formulations or regional items have not been included. This information is current as of October 2009. When checking for food allergens, please keep in mind that fried products may be cooked using shared frying oil.

Eggs and Sides:
Side Salad
Grits w/ Margarine
Original Scrambler w/ Bacon
Original Scrambler w/ Sausage
4-Carb Scrambler w/ Bacon
4-Carb Scrambler w/ Sausage
Southwestern Scrambler
Grits

Drinks:
Sour Green Apple Freeze
Grape Freeze
Strawberry Freeze
Pomegranate Freeze
Cherry Freeze
Blueberry Freeze
Banana Freeze
Coca-Cola Freeze
Blitz Energy Freeze
Blitz Energy Drink (on the rocks)
Vanilla Milkquake
Chocolate Milkquake
Strawberry Milkquake

Condiments:
Ketchup
Mustard
Mayonnaise
Apple Jelly
Grape Jelly
Strawberry Jelly
Honey
Table Syrup
Hidden Valley Ranch Dressing Cup
Ken's Steak House Sweet & Spicy Honey Mustard Dressing Cup
Ken's Steak House Cannonball barbecue Sauce Cup
Ken's Steak House Spicy Wing Sauce Cup
Hidden Valley Ranch Dressing Packet
Ken's Steak House Honey Dijon Dressing Packet
Ken's Steak House Country French with Vermont Honey Dressing Packet
Ken's Steak House Lite Italian Dressing Packet
Jalapenos

Disclaimer: We do not guarantee, nor do these restaurants guarantee that any menu item will be 100% gluten-free. These restaurants & Business Graphics Group assume no liability for your use of this information. See full disclaimer on page 7.

Legal Sea Foods

All Legal Sea Foods restaurants have a Gluten Free Menu (LTK concepts do not at this time) which also includes children's items. Legal Sea Foods regards allergy and dietary concerns very seriously. We want our Guests to dine with us in confidence. If you have an allergy or dietary concern, please ask to speak with a manager or chef when you next visit any of our restaurants. They are prepared to consult with you, offer ingredient information, work to keep your ordered items free from cross-contamination and oversee the preparation of your entire meal. Each location may have a slightly different gluten-free menu. You can search for your location here: www.legalseafoods.com. **Please be understanding of extra preparation time.**

Lunch:
Shrimp and Garlic – *no pasta*
Portuguese Fisherman's Stew – *no bread*
Grilled Shrimp
Grilled Sea Scallops
Grilled Atlantic Salmon
Crispy Sea Scallops (*request fry in chick pea flour*)
Crispy Shrimp (*request fry in chick pea flour*)
Jasmine Special
Classic Caesar Salad (*request gluten free croutons*)
Lobster Salad – *no bun*
Crabmeat Salad – *no roll*
Niman Ranch Burger – *no roll*

Seafood Bar:
Raw Oysters
Raw Littleneck Clams
Raw Cherrystone Clams
(*No cocktail sauce, it is not gluten free*)

Appetizers:
Pan Seared Raw Tuna Sashimi- *no sesame vinaigrette, no seaweed salad*
Jumbo Shrimp Cocktail – *no cocktail sauce*
Steamers
Mussels
Hot Lump Crab Dip with Seafood Chips
Crispy Montauk Calamari – *request fry in chick pea flour*

Completely Legal:
Wood Grilled Swordfish
Everything Tuna
Surf & Turf
Filet Mignon
Cioppino – *no bread*
Anna's Baked Boston Scrod – *request gluten free crumbs*
Baked Grey Sole – *request gluten free crumbs*
Wood Grilled Assortment
Shrimp and Garlic – *no pasta*
Seafood Casserole – *request gluten free crumbs, no cream sauce*
Steamed Lobsters
Baked Stuffed Lobsters – *request gluten free crumbs*
New England Lobster Bake – *no crackers*

Wood Grilled Fish:
Atlantic Salmon
Tuna
Swordfish
Rainbow Trout
Bluefish (also available crispy fried – *request chick pea flour*)
Shrimp
Sea Scallops
Haddock

Disclaimer: We do not guarantee, nor do these restaurants guarantee that any menu item will be 100% gluten-free. These restaurants & Business Graphics Group assume no liability for your use of this information. See full disclaimer on page 7.

Legal Sea Foods Continued:

Chowders, Soups & Salads:
Lite Clam Chowder – *no crackers*
Rasam Seafood Soup - *no crackers*
House Salad
Classic Caesar Salad – *request gluten free croutons*

Children's Menu:
Half Steamed Lobster
Fresh Cod Fish Sticks (*request fry in chick pea flour*)
Hamburger – *no bun*
Cheeseburger - *no bun*

Sides:
Steamed broccoli
Seasonal vegetables
Steamed snap peas
Brown rice
Jasmine rice
Baked potato

Desserts:
Belgian Chocolate Mousse Parfait
Sorbet
Seasonal Fruit

Some items that are NOT gluten free: Cocktail Sauce, Balsamic Vinaigrette, Rice Pilaf, Crackers, Bread (although some locations may have a gluten free roll), Crumbs, Clam Fry Mix, Chinese Sauces, French Fries, and Ice Cream

Gluten Sensitivity, Gluten Intolerance or Celiac Sprue Disease

People who have gluten sensitivities exclude all sources of the following grains from their diet: wheat, rye, barley, oats, spelt, and their derivatives. Legal Sea Foods has taken the necessary precautions to ensure that the following menu items and their preparations are free of elements that might cause a reaction for those with gluten sensitivity. If you have any concerns about any of these items, please consult your physician prior to trying them. For your safety, we WILL NOT substitute. All seafood and meat items will be prepared by the following methods: wood grilled, steamed, pan-seared, baked with gluten free crumbs, or fried in chick pea flour. All cookware and plateware will be pre-washed and wiped dry before cooking and presentation. These menu items require special attention, please allow us additional time to prepare your meal. A manager will consult with you and follow your order through to completion. Our goal is to provide our guests who suffer from gluten sensitivities with a menu so they may dine at Legal Sea Foods in confidence. Enjoy!

Disclaimer: We do not guarantee, nor do these restaurants guarantee that any menu item will be 100% gluten-free. These restaurants & Business Graphics Group assume no liability for your use of this information. See full disclaimer on page 7.

Logan's Roadhouse

The following information about gluten-free menu items has been obtained either from the restaurant's website or through direct contact with guest services via email or phone.

*IMMEDIATELY NOTIFY MANAGER OF GUESTS' SPECIAL ALLERGY NEEDS
DISCLAIMER: While Logan's Roadhouse strives to create a unique dining experience that positively impacts all of our guests, Logan's Roadhouse does not have a gluten-free kitchen. We will, however, make every attempt to meet your needs for a gluten-restricted diet. While the recommendations below are based on the elimination of certain ingredients from menu items and include changes in the foods preparation, Logan's Roadhouse does not guarantee that the food is prepared free of any or all allergens. The menu options below are based on the current ingredients being used at Logan's corporate owned locations and are not valid in CA, NC, SC and Augusta, GA. These suggestions are based on ingredients from our current suppliers and do not include store bought ingredients. If you have any questions regarding the menu options below or the foods preparation, please request to speak to a manager.

Appetizer:
Smokin' Hot Wings (*ask if they are fried with gluten-containing items*)

Entrée Salads:
Roadhouse Salad, Mesquite-Grilled Chicken Salad, Grilled Steak Salad, Grilled Shrimp & Veggie Skewers Salad: *DO NOT serve with croutons or bacon bits. Serve ONLY with gluten-free dressings.*

Steaks: (*ONLY these listed ones*) - The Logan, 6oz & 8oz Sirloin, 12oz & 18oz, NY Strip, 6oz, 8oz & 12oz Filet, 12oz & 16oz, Ribeye, 16oz T-Bone, 18oz Porterhouse, 20oz Ribeye, Chopped Steak (*served plain - without gravy, without mushrooms and onions*)

Burgers: *DO NOT serve with the bun.*
Mesquite-Grilled Salmon: *DO NOT serve with garlic-dill sauce.*
Santa Fe Tilapia: *DO NOT serve with tortilla strips, Roasted Corn and Black Bean salsa or Roadhouse Ranch.*
Logan's Mesquite Grilled Chicken: *DO NOT serve on a bed of rice.*
Baby Back Ribs: No changes required.
Triple Shrimp Skewers: *DO NOT serve on a bed of rice.*

Sides:
Baked Potato: *No whipped margarine.* SERVE with cubes of block butter.
Logan's Sweet Potato: *No whipped margarine.* SERVE with cubes of block butter.
Broccoli: *DO NOT use seasoned butter blend.* USE cubes of block butter with grill spice.
House Salad - SERVE only with recommended gluten-free dressings. *DO NOT serve with bacon bits.*
Grilled Vegetable / Grilled Mushroom Skewer: NO changes required

---

Disclaimer: We do not guarantee, nor do these restaurants guarantee that any menu item will be 100% gluten-free. These restaurants & Business Graphics Group assume no liability for your use of this information. See full disclaimer on page 7.

Logan's Roadhouse Continued:

Dessert: Ice Cream: NO changes required.

Gluten-Free Dressings and Seasonings: Ken's Foods: Red French dressing, bleu cheese dressing, Parmesean peppercorn dressing, honey mustard dressing, deluxe ranch dressing, balsamic vinaigrette dressing, texas petal sauce, honey bbq sauce. Kraft Foods: golden Italian marinade/dressing, thousand island dressing, classic dijon mustard (grey poupon), fat free ranch dressing, Lemon pepper - Newly wed's foods, southwest seasoning - newly wed's foods grill spice - newly wed's foods, seasoning salt – newly wed's foods, blackening seasoning – newly wed's foods, cinnamon sugar – newly wed's foods, fry seasoning – newly wed's foods, Phase – ventura Foods.

Disclaimer: We do not guarantee, nor do these restaurants guarantee that any menu item will be 100% gluten-free. These restaurants & Business Graphics Group assume no liability for your use of this information. See full disclaimer on page 7.

LongHorn Steak House

The following information about gluten-free menu items has been obtained either from the restaurant's website or through direct contact with guest services via email or phone.

Although LongHorn Steakhouse does not have a gluten-free kitchen, we will make every attempt to meet your needs for a gluten-restricted diet. The items listed on the menu below are appropriate for a gluten-restricted diet, as is, or can be ordered with minor changes (listed in italics). To insure that your meal is prepared properly, please request that all items be prepared in separate containers and on freshly cleaned food contact surfaces.

Salads:
Request NO croutons on salads.
Request that salads be tossed in separate mixing bowls from other salads.
Sonoma Chicken Salad
7-Pepper Salad
Chicken Caesar Salad
Grilled Salmon Salad- *order without Salmon Marinade*
Mixed Green Side Salad
Caesar Side Salad

Dressings: House, Ranch, Fat-free Ranch, Balsamic Vinaigrette, Thousand Island, Chipotle Ranch, Bleu Cheese, Caesar, Honey Mustard, Oil and Vinegar

Burgers/Sandwiches:
Cheese Burger -*Order without bun or French fries*
Bacon Cheese Burger- *Order without bun or French fries*
Shaved Prime Rib Sandwich -*Order without bun, horseradish sauce, or French fries*
Honey Mustard Chicken Sandwich- *Order without bun or French fries*

Ribs, Chops, Etc.:
Babyback Ribs- *order without BBQ sauce or French fries*
Cowboy Pork Chop- *order without spiced Apples or French Fries*

Seafood:
All Salmon must be ordered without the Salmon Marinade
Flo's Filet and Salmon
LongHorn Salmon
Redrock Grilled Shrimp
Flo's Filet and Lobster Tail (where available)

Chicken:
Rocky Top Chicken- *order without BBQ sauce*
Sierra Chicken

Side Items:
Baked Potato
Mashed Potatoes
Asparagus Spears
Seasonal Vegetables
Sweet Potato
Jalapeno coleslaw
Sliced Tomatoes
Grilled Onions
Sautéed Mushrooms

Kids Meals:
Kid's Hot Dog -*without bun or French fries*
Kid's Cheese Burger *without bun or French fries*
Kid's Grilled Chicken Salad- *without croutons*
Kid's Sirloin Steak- *without French Fries*
Kid's Grilled Chicken
Kid's BBQ Ribs- *without BBQ sauce or French Fries*

Disclaimer: We do not guarantee, nor do these restaurants guarantee that any menu item will be 100% gluten-free. These restaurants & Business Graphics Group assume no liability for your use of this information. See full disclaimer on page 7.

Longhorn Steak House Continued:

Legendary Steaks:
Flo's Filet
Peppered Bacon Wrapped Filet
NY Strip
LongHorn Porterhouse
Prime Rib -*Order without Classic Au Jus, French Onion Au Jus, Roasted Garlic Cream Sauce or Horseradish Sauce*
Ribeye
Renegade Top Sirloin
Fire-Grilled T-Bone
Chop Steak -*order without Mushroom Bordelaise sauce, or crisp onion straws, or French fries*

Desserts:
Hot Fudge Sundae
Fresh Fruit

Disclaimer: We do not guarantee, nor do these restaurants guarantee that any menu item will be 100% gluten-free. These restaurants & Business Graphics Group assume no liability for your use of this information. See full disclaimer on page 7.

Long John Silver's

The following information about gluten-free menu items has been obtained either from the restaurant's website or through direct contact with guest services via email or phone.

Seafood:
Grilled Pacific Salmon *(Products are prepared in common equipment and therefore may contain allergen or ingredient.)*
Shrimp Scampi *(Products are prepared in common equipment and therefore may contain allergen or ingredient.)*

Bowls:
Freshside Grille Smart Choice Salmon *(Products are prepared in common equipment and therefore may contain allergen or ingredient.)*
Freshside Grille Smart Choice Shrimp Scampi *(Products are prepared in common equipment and therefore may contain allergen or ingredient.)*

Sauces:
Cocktail Sauce
Ketchup
Louisiana Hot Sauce
Tartar Sauce
Baja Sauce
Louisiana Hot Sauce
Ketchup

Side Dishes
Coleslaw
Corn Cobbette
Corn Cobbette With Butter Oil
Vegetable Medley *(products are prepared in common equipment and therefore may contain allergen or ingredient)*
Rice

Dollar Stretcher Menu
Baja Chicken Taco

Lemonades
Regular Iceflow Lemonade
Strawberry Iceflow Lemonade

The allergen information displayed on this site is based on standard product formulations and is current as of September 30, 2009. Variations may occur due to differences in suppliers, ingredient substitutions, recipe revisions, and/or product production at the restaurant.

Disclaimer: We do not guarantee, nor do these restaurants guarantee that any menu item will be 100% gluten-free. These restaurants & Business Graphics Group assume no liability for your use of this information. See full disclaimer on page 7.

Macaroni Grill

The following information about gluten-free menu items has been obtained either from the restaurant's website or through direct contact with guest services via email or phone.

PRIOR TO PLACING YOUR ORDER, PLEASE ALWAYS ALERT THE MANAGER TO YOUR FOOD ALLERGY OR SPECIAL DIETARY NEEDS

Suggested Beverage & Menu Options for WHEAT/GLUTEN Allergies

We have prepared this suggested list of beverage and menu options based on the most current ingredient information from our food suppliers and their stated absence of wheat within these items. Please be aware that during normal kitchen operations involving shared cooking and preparation areas, including common fryer oil, the possibility exists for food items to come in contact with other food products. <u>Due to these circumstances, we are unable to guarantee that any menu entrée can be completely free of allergens.</u>

Fresh Antipasti:
(Includes sauces & garnishes)
Mediterranean Olives – *w/o Peasant Bread*
Mozzarella alla Caprese

Insalata:
(Includes dressing unless otherwise stated & *w/o croutons*)
Caesar Salad
Chicken Caesar
Fresh Greens Salad
Parmesan-Crusted Chicken w/ Grilled Chicken Breast
Scallops & Spinach Salad
Warm Spinach Salad – *w/o Goat Cheese*

Salad Dressings:
Balsamic Vinaigrette, Caesar, Mediterranean Vinaigrette, Peppercorn Ranch

Handcrafted Pasta:
Shrimp Portofino – *w/o Panko Breadcrumbs & w/o Pasta*
Sausage Salentino – *w/o Pasta*

Sides:
Grilled Asparagus, Spinach & Garlic

Mediterranean Grill:
Aged Beef Tenderloin Spiedini – *w/o Vegetables*
Calabrese Steak – *w/o Sides*
Center-Cut Filet – *w/o Sides*
Center-Cut Lamb Spiedini – *w/o Vegetables*
Grilled Chicken Spiedini – *w/o Vegetables*
Italian Sausage Spiedini – *w/o Vegetables*
Jumbo Shrimp Spiedini – *w/o Vegetables*
Grilled Halibut – *w/o Risotto*

Kid's:
Beef Kabob
Crisp Salad
Grilled Chicken & Broccoli – *w/o Pasta*
Vanilla Gelato

Dessert:
Italian Sorbetto – *w/o Biscotti*

Beverages: :
Coke, Diet Coke, Dr. Pepper, Sprite,
Italian & Italian Cream Sodas: Blackberry, Mango, Pomegranate & Sicilian Orange,
Tea: Blackberry Mint, Mango, Peach & Raspberry,
Red & White Wine

Disclaimer: We do not guarantee, nor do these restaurants guarantee that any menu item will be 100% gluten-free. These restaurants & Business Graphics Group assume no liability for your use of this information. See full disclaimer on page 7.

Macaroni Grill Continued:

At Romano's Macaroni Grill, a top priority is always the health and safety of our guests. As part of our commitment to you, our allergen menus are based on product information provided by Macaroni Grill's approved food manufacturers. Every effort is made to keep this information current. However, it is possible that ingredient changes and substitutions may occur due to the differences in regional suppliers, recipe revisions, preparation techniques, and/or the season of the year. Certain menu items may vary from restaurant to restaurant and may not be available at all locations. We highly recommend that our guests with food allergies or special dietary needs consult with a restaurant manager prior to placing an order to ensure the posted information is accurate and represents the menu items sold at that particular location. Limited time offers, test products, or regional items have not been included in the menus. Valid only through 5/1/2010 – 5/17/2010

Disclaimer: We do not guarantee, nor do these restaurants guarantee that any menu item will be 100% gluten-free. These restaurants & Business Graphics Group assume no liability for your use of this information. See full disclaimer on page 7.

Max & Erma's

The following information about gluten-free menu items has been obtained either from the restaurant's website or through direct contact with guest services via email or phone.

Due to the many ingredients that are used in our food-making process, we virtually make no guarantees regarding the presence of particular items in our menu. However, we are in the process of gathering a list of gluten-free items.

Listed below some of the items we know to be gluten-free.

Plain hamburger (no bun or toppings)

Our Laredo steak is not marinated so this would be an option, but you would have to eliminate the cactus butter.

Plain salads (please check our list of toppings on the menu). We do offer oil and vinegar dressing. Our other dressings do contain gluten.

Please note that all of our chicken items are marinated.

Our baked potatoes are coated with a soy based vegetable oil prior to baking. If soy is an issue, this would pose a problem.

Our 6 1/2 oz. sandwich chicken breast is marinated in a neutral marinade that does not contain gluten, although we do use a soy based shortening to coat the breast prior to cooking. You could request the cooks to use that particular breast and char grill it with absolutely nothing on it in order to be as safe as possible.

Disclaimer: We do not guarantee, nor do these restaurants guarantee that any menu item will be 100% gluten-free. These restaurants & Business Graphics Group assume no liability for your use of this information. See full disclaimer on page 7.

McAlister's Deli

The following information about gluten-free menu items has been obtained either from the restaurant's website or through direct contact with guest services via email or phone.

Gluten-Free Choices*

McAlister's is sensitive to the requirements of guests with gluten intolerance and we make every effort to provide options on our menu. Following is a list of gluten-free choices:

Sandwiches: (*without bread*)
Smoked Deli Turkey
Roast Beef
Corned Beef
Chicken Salad
Tuna Salad

Soup & Chili:
Southwestern Roasted Corn Soup

Spuds:
Plain Baked Potato with or without Land-O-Lakes Butter

Sides:
Mashed Potatoes without gravy
Potato Salad
Steamed Broccoli and Carrots
Fruit Salad
Fajita Chicken Strips

Dressings and Extras:
All cheeses are Gluten Free
Lite Sour Cream
All Salad Dressings are Gluten Free
Bacon
Bacon Bits

* Several of our vendors have supplied us with statements quantifying their products gluten free. Please be aware that we may change vendors and/or ingredients on a product as needed without notification. We are only able to make the above recommendations with the current vendor statements and are not liable or responsible for future menu changes. Please feel free to ask us for updated information.

** Grilled Chicken Breast is NOT Gluten Free because of the seasoning used on our sandwiches and our salads.

Disclaimer: We do not guarantee, nor do these restaurants guarantee that any menu item will be 100% gluten-free. These restaurants & Business Graphics Group assume no liability for your use of this information. See full disclaimer on page 7.

McDonalds

McDonald's no longer maintains a list of products that are considered gluten free. We do, however, provide extensive nutrition and ingredient information for our nationally offered menu product on our website. We update the information on our website frequently as we receive new information from our product suppliers. We encourage you to read our ingredient statements and make personal decisions that meet your specific dietary needs.

100% Beef Patty – *no bun*
Bacon
Ketchup
Leaf Lettuce
Lettuce
Mayonnaise Dressing
McRib Pork Patty – *no bun*
McRib Sauce
Mustard
Natural Swiss Cheese
Onions
Pasteurized Process American Cheese
Pickle Slices
Premium Ranch Sauce
Quarter Pound 100% Beef Patty
Red Onions
Sauteed Mushrooms
Shredded Cheddar/Jack Cheese
Tangy Honey Mustard Sauce
Tartar Sauce
Tomato Slice
Ketchup Packet
Honey
Hot Mustard Sauce
Spicy Buffalo Sauce
Creamy Ranch Sauce
Sausage Patty
Scrambled Eggs
Bacon
Breakfast Steak
Canadian Style Bacon
Egg
Folded Egg
Pasteurized Process American Cheese
Potato Vegetable Blend
Salsa Roja
Sausage & Scrambled Egg Mix
Shredded Cheddar/Jack Cheese
Slivered Onions

Salads:
Premium Southwest Salad (*without chicken and no croutons*)
Premium Bacon Ranch Salad (*without chicken and no croutons*)
Premium Caesar Salad (*without chicken and no croutons*)
Side Salad (*no croutons*)
Bacon Bits

Salad Dressings
Newman's Own® Creamy Southwest Dressing
Newman's Own® Creamy Caesar Dressing
Newman's Own® Low Fat Balsamic Vinaigrette
Newman's Own® Low Fat Family Recipe Italian Dressing
Newman's Own® Ranch

Desserts/Shakes:
Fruit 'n Yogurt Parfait (*without granola*)
Low Fat Caramel Dip
Strawberry Sundae
Hot Caramel Sundae
Hot Fudge Sundae
Peanuts (for Sundaes)

Iced Coffee-- Caramel
Iced Coffee-- Hazelnut
Iced Coffee-- Regular
Iced Coffee-- Vanilla
Iced Coffee with Sugar Free Vanilla Syrup
Sweet Tea
Nonfat Cappuccino
Nonfat Latte
Nonfat Caramel Cappuccino
Nonfat Caramel Latte
Iced Nonfat Caramel Latte
Iced Nonfat Hazelnut Latte
Iced Nonfat Vanilla Latte
Iced Nonfat Latte
Latte with Sugar Free Vanilla Syrup
Cappuccino
Latte
Caramel Cappuccino
Caramel Latte
Hazelnut Cappuccino
Hazelnut Latte
Vanilla Cappuccino
Vanilla Latte
Cappuccino with Sugar Free Vanilla Syrup
Latte with Sugar Free Vanilla Syrup
Mocha
Hot Chocolate
Iced Latte
Iced Caramel Latte

Disclaimer: We do not guarantee, nor do these restaurants guarantee that any menu item will be 100% gluten-free. These restaurants & Business Graphics Group assume no liability for your use of this information. See full disclaimer on page 7.

McDonalds Continued

McFlurry® with M&M'S® Candies
Apple Dippers with Low Fat Caramel Dip
Chocolate McCafé® Shake
Chocolate Triple Thick® Shake
Strawberry Banana Smoothie
Strawberry Banana Smoothie without Yogurt
Strawberry McCafé® Shake
Strawberry Triple Thick® Shake
Vanilla McCafé® Shake
Vanilla Triple Thick® Shake
Wild Berry Smoothie
Wild Berry Smoothie without Yogurt
Nonfat Hazelnut Cappuccino
Nonfat Hazelnut Latte
Nonfat Vanilla Cappuccino
Nonfat Vanilla Latte
Nonfat Cappuccino with
Iced Hazelnut Latte
Iced Vanilla Latte
Iced Latte with Sugar Free Vanilla Syrup
Iced Mocha
McCafe Frappes
Frappe Caramel
Frappe Mocha
Sugar Free Vanilla Syrup
Nonfat Latte with Sugar Free Vanilla Syrup
Mocha with Nonfat Milk
Hot Chocolate with Nonfat Milk
Iced Nonfat Latte

This list is effective 06-03-2010. The nutrition information on this website is derived from testing conducted in accredited laboratories, published resources, or from information provided from McDonald's suppliers. The nutrition information is based on standard product formulations and serving sizes. All nutrition information is based on average values for ingredients from McDonald's suppliers throughout the U.S. and is rounded to meet current US FDA NLEA guidelines. Variation in serving sizes, preparation techniques, product testing and sources of supply, as well as regional and seasonal differences may affect the nutrition values for each product. In addition, product formulations change periodically. You should expect some variation in the nutrient content of the products purchased in our restaurants. None of our products is certified as vegetarian. This information is correct as of January 2007, unless stated otherwise.

Disclaimer: We do not guarantee, nor do these restaurants guarantee that any menu item will be 100% gluten-free. These restaurants & Business Graphics Group assume no liability for your use of this information. See full disclaimer on page 7.

Melting Pot

The following information about gluten-free menu items has been obtained either from the restaurant's website or through direct contact with guest services via email or phone.

Cheese Fondue: *request a GF cheese dipper bowl and no bread or chips*
Spinach Artichoke Cheese Fondue *(request to be made with cornstarch)*
Wisconsin Trio Cheese Fondue *(request to be made with cornstarch)*
Fiesta Cheese Fondue *(request to be made with cornstarch and Redbridge® beer)*
Cheddar Cheese Fondue *(request to be made with cornstarch and Redbridge® beer)*
Traditional Swiss Cheese Fondue *(request to be made with cornstarch)*

Salads:
The Melting Pot House Salad *(request no croutons)*
Spinach Mushroom Salad
Caesar Salad *(request no croutons)*
California Salad

Individual Entrée Selections
Land & Sea
The French Quarter
Seafood Trio
Cedar Plank Salmon
Breast of Chicken
Signature Selection *(Request a substitution for teriyaki-marinated sirloin)*
Pacific Rim *(Request a substitution for teriyaki-marinated sirloin and potstickers)*
The Vegetarian *(Request substitutions for tofu, ravioli and pasta, request no batters)*
Filet Mignon
Add Lobster Tail

Entrée Cooking Styles:
Coq au Vin
Court Bouillon
Bourguignon *(request no batters)*
Mojo Style
Entrée Sauces:
Curry
Green Goddess
Gorgonzola Port
Ginger Plum

Chocolate Fondue: *Request GF dessert plate: strawberries, bananas, plain marshmallows and pineapple*
Big Night Out Chocolate – Passion Fruit Yin & Yang Fondue
The Original
Bananas Foster
DISARRONO® Meltdown
Yin & Yang
Cookies 'n Cream Marshmallow Dream *(request no crushed Oreo cookies)*
Chocolate S'mores *(request no crushed graham crackers)*
Flaming Turtle
Pure Chocolate
Special Event

Disclaimer: We do not guarantee, nor do these restaurants guarantee that any menu item will be 100% gluten-free. These restaurants & Business Graphics Group assume no liability for your use of this information. See full disclaimer on page 7.

Mitchell's Fish Market

The following information about gluten-free menu items has been obtained either from the restaurant's website or through direct contact with guest services via email or phone.

This menu and all of the information on it is provided by Mitchell's Fish Market, in cooperation with the Gluten Intolerance Group (GIG), as a service to our guests. Mitchell's Fish Market and GIG assume no responsibility for its use and any resulting liability or consequential damages is denied. Cynthia Kupper, a Registered Dietician with GIG, prepared this information (which has not been verified by Mitchell's Fish Market).

Guests are encouraged to consider this information in light of their individual requirements and needs. GIG extends our sincere appreciation to Mitchell's Fish Market Restaurants for being proactive by making it easier for persons with gluten intolerances to enjoy dining out.

Appetizers:
Pan Roasted Wild Blue Mussels ~ *REQUEST NO CROUTONS*
Seared Hawaiian Ahi Tuna ~ *REQUEST NO SAUCES OR CRACKERS*
Oysters & Raw Bar ~ *REQUEST NO CRACKERS*
Today's Oyster Selections
Louisiana Style Charbroiled Oysters ~ *REQUEST NO BREAD*

Salads:
All our dressings are gluten free
"Titanic" Wedge of Iceberg
The Market's Famous House Salad
Our Classic Caesar ~ *REQUEST NO CROUTONS* With grilled marinated chicken breast, Grilled salmon or spicy grilled shrimp
Spinach Salad
Blackened Salmon Spinach Salad
Grilled Harpoon Shrimp Salad

Today's Fresh Catch:
All Fresh Catch Species are gluten free and can be prepared
any of the ways listed below; please see menu for daily selections
Shang Hai ~ *REQUEST NO RICE WINE SAUCE*
Simply Grilled or Broiled
Blackened ~ *REQUEST NO ETOUFFEE*

Specialties & Combinations:
"House Specialty" Cedar Plank Salmon
Grilled Shrimp and Scallops Skewers ~ *REQUEST NO FLOUR*
Shang Hai Seafood Sampler ~ *REQUEST NO RICE WINE SAUCE*
The Fish Market Trio ~ *REQUEST NO ETOUFFEE OR RICE WINE SAUCE*

Disclaimer: We do not guarantee, nor do these restaurants guarantee that any menu item will be 100% gluten-free. These restaurants & Business Graphics Group assume no liability for your use of this information. See full disclaimer on page 7.

Mitchell's Fish Market Continued:

Steaks & Shellfish:
Filet Mignon
Maple-Bourbon Glazed Pork Chop
Grilled Chicken Breast
Cold Water Rock Lobster Tail
Live Maine Lobster
Alaskan Red King Crab Legs
Oscar Style

Desserts:
Mini Creme Brulee ~ macerated strawberries or Daily Sorbet ~ ask your server for availability

---

Disclaimer: We do not guarantee, nor do these restaurants guarantee that any menu item will be 100% gluten-free. These restaurants & Business Graphics Group assume no liability for your use of this information. See full disclaimer on page 7.

Moe's Southwest Grill

The following information about gluten-free menu items has been obtained either from the restaurant's website or through direct contact with guest services via email or phone.

Moe's Southwest Grill and its franchisees and employees do not assume responsibility for a particular sensitivity or allergy to any food product provided in any Moe's Southwest Grill.

Fish
Ground Beef
Tofu
Pork
Black Beans
Pinto Beans
Black Olives
Cheese
Chipotle Ranch
Cucumbers
Guacamole
Jalapenos
Lettuce
Queso (cheese sauce)
Rice
Salsa (Kaiser & El Guapo)
Sour Cream
Southwest Vinaigrette
Veggies
Tomatillo Salsa
Pico De Gallo
Hard Rock Sauce
Rock 'N Roll Sauce
Baja Chicken Enchilada Soup

the wraps and chips are not gluten-free

Disclaimer: We do not guarantee, nor do these restaurants guarantee that any menu item will be 100% gluten-free. These restaurants & Business Graphics Group assume no liability for your use of this information. See full disclaimer on page 7.

Morton's The Steakhouse

The following information about gluten-free menu items has been obtained either from the restaurant's website or through direct contact with guest services via email or phone.

Morton's The Steakhouse does not have a specific gluten free menu, however, we do have many menu options that are gluten free, including some salads, entrees including steaks, as long as you don't order the seasoning or sauces that accompany them.

We offer fresh fruit as an alternative for dessert. Your sever will be able to provide recommendations in order to avoid anything you may be allergic to.

If you need to make special arrangements ahead of time you may call the location directly that you are going to visit and speak with the General Manager who can arrange something with the chef as well inform the kitchen to take special precautions when preparing your meal.

Disclaimer: We do not guarantee, nor do these restaurants guarantee that any menu item will be 100% gluten-free. These restaurants & Business Graphics Group assume no liability for your use of this information. See full disclaimer on page 7.

Ninety-Nine Restaurants

The following information about gluten-free menu items has been obtained either from the restaurant's website or through direct contact with guest services via email or phone.

Please inform your server of any dietary concerns. Your best source for health information and guidance is your physician. Please don't take this menu as medical advice. It is an informational resource only, and we are not responsible for how you use this information. Consult your physician if you have questions about whether certain foods may cause allergic reactions. We take great care to ensure the foods offered on this menu are free of gluten and gluten derivatives, but we are not responsible for individual reactions to any foods and cannot guarantee that the foods we serve are allergen-free. *Cooked to order. "Consuming raw or undercooked meats, poultry, seafood, shellfish or eggs may increase your risk of food borne illness, especially if you have certain medical conditions.© Ninety Nine Restaurants T1 4/10"

Fresh From The Garden:
Caesar Salad: *Please order without croutons and Rustic Bread*
Chicken Caesar Salad: *Please order without Rustic Bread and croutons*
Garden Salad: *Please order without croutons*

Dressing Options: Bleu Cheese, Buttermilk Ranch, Honey Mustard, Northern Italian,

Guest Inspired Chef Created:
Prime Rib *Please order without au jus*
Broiled Sirloin Tips
Smothered Tips
NY Strip Sirloin
Top Sirloin Steak
Cedar Plank Salmon

Combo Creations: *Please order without honey butter biscuit*
Kickin' Shrimp Skewer
Top Sirloin Steak
Cedar Plank Salmon

Classic Sides:
Garlic Red Skin Mashed Potatoes
Baked Potato
Load a Mashed Potato with Cheese, Bacon & Chives
French Fries (*where available – confirm that they are fried in a dedicated fryer*)
Seasonal Vegetables

Two Hands Required: Gluten Free Roll is available!
Bacon & Cheese Steakburger: *Ask for a Gluten-Free Roll*
Mushroom & Cheese Steakburger: *Ask for a Gluten-Free Roll*
All Star Steakburger: *Ask for a Gluten-Free Roll*

Kid's Menu:
Junior Top Sirloin Steak
Junior Steakburger with Cheese: *Ask for a Gluten-Free Roll*

Irresistible Endings:
Ice Cream Sundae

Disclaimer: We do not guarantee, nor do these restaurants guarantee that any menu item will be 100% gluten-free. These restaurants & Business Graphics Group assume no liability for your use of this information. See full disclaimer on page 7.

Noodles & Company

The following information about gluten-free menu items has been obtained either from the restaurant's website or through direct contact with guest services via email or phone.

Watching Gluten?

We sell noodles, and a lot of them, so we can't guarantee that your food won't come into contact with gluten, but we will do our best to accommodate your request. So if you're looking to reduce gluten, try these dishes with rice noodles. There is no gluten in the ingredients:

Penne Rosa with rice noodles
Pesto Cavatappi with rice noodles
Pasta Fresca with rice noodles
Tuscan Linguine with rice noodles
Spaghetti with marinara sauce with rice noodles
Buttered Noodles with rice noodles

Here are some other dishes you also might try:

Pad Thai
Chinese Chop Salad with fat-free Asian dressing and no wonton strips
The Med Salad with no cavatappi noodles
Caesar Salad with no croutons
Tossed Green Side Salad with fat-free Asian dressing
Cucumber Tomato Side Salad

Of Interest: We have peanuts, tree nuts, soy, milk, eggs, fish, shellfish and wheat in our restaurant, and there may be cross contact with your food. In addition, because we offer so many unique flavors, not every ingredient we use is listed in our menu descriptions.

We periodically update this guide. We also test new dishes or change suppliers and may not be able to reflect such changes within this guide.

*Ask to see if they cook the rice noodles in the same water/pots as they do the "regular" noodles to be sure they are gluten-free.

Disclaimer: We do not guarantee, nor do these restaurants guarantee that any menu item will be 100% gluten-free. These restaurants & Business Graphics Group assume no liability for your use of this information. See full disclaimer on page 7.

The Old Spaghetti Factory

The following information about gluten-free menu items has been obtained either from the restaurant's website or through direct contact with guest services via email or phone.

Gluten-Free Options

Salad:
House Salad – *Request no croutons* (Add Chicken also available)

Dressing:
Balsamic Vinaigrette
Creamy Pesto

Entrees:
Gluten Free Rice Fettuccini (Add Italian Sausage or chicken breast)

Sauce Options:
Marinara Sauce
Rich Meat Sauce
Sautéed Mushroom Sauce
Mizithra Cheese & Browned Butter

Baked Chicken (with side of Gluten Free Rice Fettuccine with above sauce options)

Beverages:
Italian Cream Soda
Strawberry Lemonade
Soft Drinks
Coffee, Tea, Iced Tea or Milk

Desserts:
Ice Cream: Vanilla, Spumoni

Disclaimer: We do not guarantee, nor do these restaurants guarantee that any menu item will be 100% gluten-free. These restaurants & Business Graphics Group assume no liability for your use of this information. See full disclaimer on page 7.

Olive Garden

The following information about gluten-free menu items has been obtained either from the restaurant's website or through direct contact with guest services via email or phone.

While Olive Garden has made an effort to provide complete and current gluten content information, changes in recipes, and the hand crafted nature of our menu items, mean that variations in the ingredient profile of a particular menu item may occur from time to time. Guests with gluten intolerance or other special food sensitivities should not rely solely on this information. Olive Garden assumes no liability for your use of this information. Any medical concerns regarding the consumption of these items should be directed to your physician or other health care provider. If you would like to speak with an Olive Garden representative, please call us at 800-331-2729.

Salads:
Garden Salad - order without croutons
Caesar Salad - order without croutons

Entrees:
Pennine Rigate with Marinara - served over a gluten-free penne pasta
Steak Toscano
Herb-Grilled Salmon
Mixed Grill - skewers of grilled steak and chicken marinated in Italian herbs and extra-virgin olive oil and served with broccoli and grilled vegetables. (*please ask that it be served without the demi-glaze*)
Mixed Grill with Chicken only - skewers of chicken marinated in Italian herbs and extra-virgin olive oil and served with broccoli and grilled vegetables (*please ask that it be served without the demi-glaze*)

Children's Grilled Chicken - grilled chicken breast served with broccoli and grilled vegetables

The new gluten-free pasta entree is available at all locations, and yes, it is prepared separately to avoid cross-introduction.

Disclaimer: We do not guarantee, nor do these restaurants guarantee that any menu item will be 100% gluten-free. These restaurants & Business Graphics Group assume no liability for your use of this information. See full disclaimer on page 7.

On The Border Mexican Grill

We have prepared this suggested list of beverage and menu options based on the most current ingredient information from our food suppliers and their stated absence of wheat/gluten within these items. Please be aware that during normal kitchen operations involving shared cooking and preparation areas, including common fryer oil, the possibility exists for food items to come in contact with other food products. Due to these circumstances, we are unable to guarantee that any menu entrée can be completely free of allergens.

Suggested Beverage & Menu Options for WHEAT/GLUTEN Allergies

Appetizers:
(All Listed W/O Tortilla Chips/Crisps & Garnish)
Guacamole & Guacamole Live,
Shaken Margarita Shrimp Cocktail

Soups & Salads:
(All Listed W/O Dressing, Tortilla Strips)
Citrus Chipotle Chicken Salad
House Salad
Sizzling Fajita Salad: Chicken or Steak *w/o Sour Cream and w/o Onions*

Salad Dressings:
Chipotle Honey Mustard, Fat Free Mango Citrus Vinaigrette, Smoked Jalapeño Vinaigrette

Fajita Grill:
(All Listed W/O Condiments, Onions, Flour Tortillas)
Fajitas: Grilled Vegetable w/Portobello Mushrooms *(Not Classic Veggies)*
Mesquite-grilled Chicken
Mesquite-grilled Steak
Pork Carnita
Veggies: El Diablo
Sauces: Chipotle Honey, Tequila Lime Chile

Fresh Grill:
Chicken Salsa Fresca
Tomatillo Chicken

OTB Taco Stand: *(All Listed W/O Sides)*
Street-Style (Mini): Chicken or Steak**Sides:**
Black Beans
Black Bean & Corn Salsa
Cilantro Lime Rice
Corn Tortilla
Guacamole
House Vegetables
Mexican Rice
Mixed Cheese
Pico
Refried Beans *w/o Blue Corn Chip*

Sauces:
Salsa, Tomato Salsa Fresca

Kids:
(All Listed W/O Sides)
Kids Grilled Chicken Entrée
Kids House Salad *w/o Dressing*
Kids Mixed Vegetables
Kids Dessert: Strawberry Sundae

Beverages:
Borderita Grande, Coke, Cuervo Paradise Rita, Diet Coke, Dr. Pepper, House Margarita, Iced Tea, Mango Passion Fruit Swirl Margarita, Milagro Agave Rita, Mojito, Perfect Patron, Red & White Wine, Sangria, Sangria Swirl Margarita, Shaken Margarita, Skinny Margaritas: Fresh Lime & Wild Berry, Sprite, Strawberry Lemonade, Watermelon Margarita

---

Disclaimer: We do not guarantee, nor do these restaurants guarantee that any menu item will be 100% gluten-free. These restaurants & Business Graphics Group assume no liability for your use of this information. See full disclaimer on page 7.

On the Border Continued:

Valid only June 1 – 30, 2010: At On The Border, a top priority is always the health and safety of our guests. As part of our commitment to you, our allergen menus are based on product information provided by On The Border's approved food manufacturers. Every effort is made to keep this information current. However, it is possible that ingredient changes and substitutions may occur due to the differences in regional suppliers, recipe revisions, preparation techniques, and/or the season of the year. Certain menu items may vary from restaurant to restaurant and may not be available at all locations. We highly recommend that our guests with food allergies or special dietary needs consult with a restaurant manager prior to placing an order to ensure the posted information is accurate and represents the menu items sold at that particular location. Limited time offers, test products, or regional items have not been included in the menus.

Disclaimer: We do not guarantee, nor do these restaurants guarantee that any menu item will be 100% gluten-free. These restaurants & Business Graphics Group assume no liability for your use of this information. See full disclaimer on page 7.

Outback Steakhouse

Aussie-Tizers® to Share:
Seared Ahi Tuna *(Avoid both dressings)*
Grilled Shrimp on the Barbie

Salads: *All salad dressings are GF, except Mustard Vinaigrette and Blue Cheese dressing. Request no croutons on salads. Request salads be mixed in a separate bowl from other salads.*
FiletWedge Salad (Roasted Filet based on availability) *Avoid Blue Cheese dressing.*
Chicken or Shrimp Caesar Salad *-no croutons.*
Queensland Salad *-no croutons.*

Outback Favorites: *Aussie Fries are not GF. Order veggies without seasonings or substitute with baked potato.*
Alice Springs Chicken®
Baby Back Ribs
Grilled Chicken on the Barbie
New Zealand Rack of Lamb: *Avoid the Cabernet sauce.*
Filet with Wild Mushroom Sauce (based on availability): *Avoid the Wild Mushroom sauce. Order veggies without seasonings.*
Sweet Glazed Roasted Pork Tenderloin: *Avoid crunchy crumb topping. Order French green beans or veggies without seasonings or substitute with baked potato.*

Signature Steaks:
Victoria's Filet®: *Avoid Blue Cheese or horseradish crumb crust.*
Outback Special®
Rib eye
New York Strip
The Melbourne
Prime Rib (based on availability): *Avoid au jus.*

Straight from the Sea: *Order veggies without seasonings or substitute with baked potato.*
Atlantic Salmon
Lobster Tails (limited markets)
Alaskan King Crab (limited markets)

Burgers & Sandwiches:
****AVOID THE BREAD and Aussie Fries. Order veggies without seasonings or substitute with baked potato.*
The Bloomin' Burger™ *Avoid Bloomin' Onion Petals.*
The Outbacker Burger
Bacon Cheese Burger
Grilled Chicken & Swiss Sandwich
Bacon, mayonnaise, mustard, ketchup, cheeses, BBQ sauce, pickles, and honey mustard sauce are all gluten free.

Freshly Made Sides:
Garlic Mashed Potatoes
Dressed Baked Potato
Sweet Potato
Fresh Seasonal Veggies *Request without seasonings*

Signature Side Salads:
House Salad
Caesar Salad
Classic Blue Cheese Wedge Salad: *Avoid blue cheese dressing.*
All salad dressings are GF, except the Mustard Vinaigrette and Blue Cheese dressing. Be sure to request no croutons and request salad be mixed in a separate bowl from other salads.

Disclaimer: We do not guarantee, nor do these restaurants guarantee that any menu item will be 100% gluten-free. These restaurants & Business Graphics Group assume no liability for your use of this information. See full disclaimer on page 7.

Outback Continued:

Add On Mates:
Grilled Scallops: *Avoid Lemon Pepper Butter Sauce.*
Lobster Tail (limited markets)
1/2 lb. Alaskan King Crab (limited markets)
Shrimp Scampi *Avoid garlic toast*
Grilled Shrimp

Perfect Combinations:
Ribs & Alice Springs Chicken®: *Aussie Fries are not GF. Order veggies without seasonings or substitute with baked potato.*
Filet & Shrimp Scampi: *Avoid garlic toast and au jus*

After-Dinner Drinks:
Grand Marnier Straight Up, Kahlúa and Coffee, DISARRONO Amaretto on the Rocks

Irresistible Desserts:
Chocolate Thunder From Down Under® This is a flourless brownie; we even dust the pan with sugar!

Joey Menu:
Aussie Fries are not GF Order veggies without seasonings or substitute with baked potato
Boomerang Cheese Burger (*no bun*)
Joey Sirloin
Grilled Chicken on the Barbie
Junior Ribs
Spotted Dog Sundae (*No Oreo crumbles*)

Outback Specialty Cocktails:
Drink selections may vary by location: Top Shelf Patrón Margarita, Sangria 'Rita, The Gold Coast 'Rita®, Captain's Mai Tai, Down Under Sauza Gold Coast 'Rita, The Wallaby Darned®, New South Wales Sangria

This menu and the information on it is provided by Outback Steakhouse, in cooperation with the Gluten Intolerance Group® (GIG®), as a service to our customers. Outback Steakhouse and GIG® assume no responsibility for its use and information which has not been verified by Outback Steakhouse. Patrons are encouraged to their own satisfaction, to consider this information in light of their individual requirements and needs. Updated 04/2010. Items may vary by location. www.gluten.net

---

Disclaimer: We do not guarantee, nor do these restaurants guarantee that any menu item will be 100% gluten-free. These restaurants & Business Graphics Group assume no liability for your use of this information. See full disclaimer on page 7.

Panera Bread

The following information about gluten-free menu items has been obtained either from the restaurant's website or through direct contact with guest services via email or phone.

Below a list of our menu items that do not contain gluten-containing ingredients. However, because we bake fresh bread daily in our bakery-cafes and bread is core to our menu, we simply cannot ensure that there has been no contact between these items, or any other menu items, and gluten.
**Although we try to meet your special requirements, we cannot ensure that these items have not come into contact with gluten in our bakery-café.

** Gorgonzola and bleu cheeses are commonly made with mold incubated on wheat. Some may choose to avoid these cheeses for this reason and you may substitute another cheese if you prefer. Items containing these ingredients are indicated below with (G) or (BC).

Salads: (including the salad dressing - source of modified food starch is corn)
- Greek Salad Fandango Salad (G)
- Caesar Salad (*without croutons*)
- Grilled Chicken Caesar Salad (*without croutons*)
- Mediterranean Salmon Salad Salmon Caesar Salad (*without croutons*)
- Asian Sesame Chicken Salad (*without Won Ton noodles*)
- Classic Cafe Salad
- Strawberry Poppyseed Salad
- Strawberry Poppyseed Salad with Chicken
- Fuji Apple Chicken Salad (G)
- California Mission Chicken Salad
- Orchard Harvest Chicken Salad (G)
- Chopped Chicken Cobb Salad (G)
- BBQ Chopped Chicken Salad

Soups:
- Low Fat Vegetarian Black Bean
- Cuban Black Bean and Lentil
- Vegetarian Roasted Red Pepper & Lentil
- Vegetarian Butternut Squash
- Creamy Tomato (*without croutons*)
- Low-Fat Vegetarian
- Southwest Tomato & Roasted Corn
- Turkey Chickpea Chili
- Summer Corn Chowder
- Low-Fat Chicken Tortilla Soup

Salad Dressings:
- Balsamic Vinaigrette
- Caesar
- Greek
- Poppyseed
- Raspberry Vinaigrette
- Asian Sesame Vinaigrette
- White Balsamic Vinaigrette
- Roasted Garlic & Meyer's
- Lemon Vinaigrette BBQ Ranch

Beverages:
- Coffee
- Juice, both apple and orange
- Lemonade
- Milk
- Soda, fountain and bottled
- Tea, regular and Chai Tea
- All lattes & Frozen beverages
- Strawberry Smoothie
- Hot Chocolate
- Pumpkin Spice Latte
- Gingerbread Latte

Panera Bread Potato Chips

Disclaimer: We do not guarantee, nor do these restaurants guarantee that any menu item will be 100% gluten-free. These restaurants & Business Graphics Group assume no liability for your use of this information. See full disclaimer on page 7.

Panera Continued:

Not all of the items listed are currently on our menu and some new menu items have not yet been evaluated for the purposes of inclusion on this list. However, you can find complete ingredients listings for current menu items on our website. (When you choose a menu item in our online Nutrition Calculator, click on the "ingredients" link for ingredients information for that item.) Please note that nutritional information on our website is updated periodically. New products may be available in our bakery-cafes before a periodic update of this site. In addition, some menu items may be available only on a regional, test or seasonal basis. Nutritional information about these menu items is available at the participating bakery-cafes. Tests of new recipes of existing products may be conducted from time to time in certain markets. These new recipes may contain different/additional ingredients, including allergens, as compared to the original version. Nutritional information about these menu items is available at the participating bakery-cafes. For the most update-to-date information, please call or visit your nearest bakery-cafe to speak with a manager.

Disclaimer: We do not guarantee, nor do these restaurants guarantee that any menu item will be 100% gluten-free. These restaurants & Business Graphics Group assume no liability for your use of this information. See full disclaimer on page 7.

Pei Wei Asian Diner

The following information about gluten-free menu items has been obtained either from the restaurant's website or through direct contact with guest services via email or phone.

Note: Products containing gluten are prepared in our kitchens.

RECOMMENDATIONS FOR GLUTEN INTOLERANT DIETS: The following items do not contain wheat, barley, rye or oats when ordered with the following preparations.

Edamame: (*cook in water, not vegetable stock*)

Vietnamese Chicken Salad Rolls: (*order without Thai peanut sauce*)

Asian Chopped Chicken Salad: (*substitute lime vinaigrette dressing and no wonton strips*)

Pei Wei Spicy Chicken Salad: (shrimp can be substituted)

Pei Wei Spicy: (choice of chicken or shrimp)

Pei Wei Sweet & Sour: (*choice of non-battered chicken or shrimp*)

Disclaimer: We do not guarantee, nor do these restaurants guarantee that any menu item will be 100% gluten-free. These restaurants & Business Graphics Group assume no liability for your use of this information. See full disclaimer on page 7.

P.F. Chang's China Bistro

The following information about gluten-free menu items has been obtained either from the restaurant's website or through direct contact with guest services via email or phone.

Notes about this Menu: These menu items are either gluten free as prepared, or are modified to be gluten free. P.F. Chang's Gluten Free Sauce contains garlic, ginger, rice wine, water, Sichuan powder, salt, sugar and wheat free soy sauce. The marinades for chicken, shrimp, scallops and calamari are gluten free and contain cornstarch. The soy sauce on the table is not gluten free. Please ask your server for our gluten free soy sauce. Products containing gluten are prepared in our kitchens.

Before placing your order, please inform your server if a person in your party has a food allergy. Additionally, if a person in your party has a special dietary need (e.g., gluten intolerance), please inform your server at the beginning or your visit. We will do our best to accommodate your needs. Please be aware that our restaurants use ingredients that contain all the major FDA allergens (peanuts, tree nuts, eggs, fish, shellfish, milk, soy and wheat).

Gluten Free Chang's Chicken Lettuce Wraps
Gluten Free Cantonese Shrimp or Scallops
Gluten Free Hong King Beef with Snow Peas
Egg Drop Soup
Gluten Free Shrimp with Lobster Sauce
Gluten Free Singapore Street Noodles
Gluten Free Chang's Spicy Chicken
Gluten Free Shrimp with Lobster Sauce Lunch Bowl
Gluten Free Fried Rice
Gluten Free Ginger Chicken with Broccoli
Gluten Free Mongolian Beef
Gluten Free Buddha's Feast
Gluten Free Philip's Better Lemon Chicken
Gluten Free Beef & Broccoli
Gluten Free Buddha's Feast Lunch Bowl
Gluten Free Moo Goo Gai Pan
Gluten Free Beef & Broccoli Lunch Bowl
Gluten Free Spinach with Garlic
Gluten Free Dali Chicken
Gluten Free Beef A La Sichuan
Gluten Free Garlic Snap Peas
Gluten Free Moo Goo Gai Pan Lunch Bowl
Gluten Free Pepper Steak
Gluten Free Shanghai Cucumbers
Gluten Free Chang's Lemon Scallops
Gluten Free Pepper Steak Lunch Bowl
Gluten Free Salmon Steamed with Ginger
GF Chocolate Dome Dessert

Disclaimer: We do not guarantee, nor do these restaurants guarantee that any menu item will be 100% gluten-free. These restaurants & Business Graphics Group assume no liability for your use of this information. See full disclaimer on page 7.

Pizza Fusion:

The following information about gluten-free menu items has been obtained either from the restaurant's website or through direct contact with guest services via email or phone.

Gluten Free Menu:
Gluten free pizza
Gluten free brownies
Gluten free beer

Pizza Fusion was created in the best interest of the individual and the environment. When originally designing the menu, Vaughan Lazar and Michael Gordon, founders of Pizza Fusion, wanted everyone to enjoy the good taste of their delicious food. So they did their research and sought out tasty alternatives that'd allow individuals with food allergies, selective diets and digestive intolerances to indulge at Pizza Fusion. The end result was a menu to be enjoyed by all that has made us especially popular amongst our vegan, vegetarian, gluten-free and lactose intolerant friends alike.

Gluten-Free Pizza
We cater to many customers with gluten intolerance with our gluten-free crust. We use a mixture of garbanzo bean, fava bean and rice flour to make our gluten-free pizza crust, and our sauce and cheese are gluten-free as well. Our gluten-free friends are always happy to know that they can order almost any topping, excluding only barbeque sauce and sausage. Our gluten-free pizza is one of the best on the market. Its great taste is a reflection of our dedication to using quality ingredients and spending the time and energy to perfect our products.

We also serve a variety of salads and melt-in-your-mouth gluten-free brownies to accompany your gluten-free pizza, as well as offer a gluten-free beer made from Sorghum instead of barley. There are many options at Pizza Fusion that fit the special dietary needs of the gluten-free community.* Our Gluten-Free crust contains the following ingredients: Bean Flour, Rice Flour, Tapioca Flour and Starch, Xanthan Gum, Salt, Yeast, Egg, Cider Vinegar, Sugar, Canola Oil, Calcium Propionate.

Vegan & Vegetarian Options
We proudly offer a truly vegan soy cheese that is casein-free to accompany our wide variety of organic veggie toppings. Our sauce is always vegan and our doughs, excluding gluten-free, are vegan, as well. We make vegetarian wraps and sandwiches, salads, and breadsticks, and we have vegan brownies for dessert that are oh so good!

Lactose-Free Cheese
Our vegan cheese is dairy and casein-free, making it a tasty option for those with lactose intolerance or anyone looking to cut dairy out of their diet. It is soy-based, and we get rave reviews from adults and kids alike on its great taste.

Disclaimer: We do not guarantee, nor do these restaurants guarantee that any menu item will be 100% gluten-free. These restaurants & Business Graphics Group assume no liability for your use of this information. See full disclaimer on page 7.

Potbelly Sandwich Shop

The following information about gluten-free menu items has been obtained either from the restaurant's website or through direct contact with guest services via email or phone.

At Potbelly Sandwich Shops food is served that may cause allergic reactions (including eggs, milk, peanuts, seafood, shellfish, soy, tree nuts, and wheat). Great care is taken to keep allergy-causing food separate from food that does not or rarely causes allergies; however, we do not guarantee any of our food to be "allergen-free." Also, our food suppliers may change ingredients that may change the information provided here. So please check back from time to time for updates. If you have a food allergy, notify the Potbelly Shop Manager BEFORE ORDERING! To learn more about food allergies, The Food Allergy and Anaphylaxis Network website at www.foodallergy.org is an excellent reference. We also recommend you consult your physician BEFORE dining with us, if you are concerned that any food at Potbelly may cause you adverse health effects. If you need ingredient lists for specific food items because you have a food allergy not addressed in this list, please e-mail us and ask through our "Talk To Us" link.

Items with no gluten declared: This means our suppliers have not listed this as a primary ingredient in their list of ingredients.

Meats & Other Sandwich "Main Stuff":
Turkey Breast
Italian Meat – Salami
Italian Meat – Capicolla
Italian Meat – Mortadello
Italian Meat – Pepperoni
Smoked Ham
Grilled Chicken
Roast Beef
Mushrooms
Marinara
Peanut Butter
Jelly
Bacon
Sausage
Egg
Swiss Cheese
Provolone Cheese
American Cheese

Sandwiches Toppings:
Mayo, Mustard, Hot Peppers (in oil)
Iceberg Lettuce, Tomatoes, Onions
Pickles, Oil

Salad Stuff:
Leafy Green Salad Blend (Romaine & Iceberg), Cucumbers, Cherry Tomatoes
Hard Boiled Egg, Blue Cheese, Chick Peas

Salad Dressings:
Buttermilk Ranch
Creamy Vinaigrette
Roasted Garlic Vinaigrette
Non-Fat Vinaigrette
Soups:
Garden Vegetable
Side Salads:
Coleslaw
Potato Salad

Shakes & Smoothies:
Chocolate, Vanilla, Strawberry Banana, Pineapple-Coconut, Boysenberry, Coffee, Mocha Dreamsickle

*Note, the bread contains gluten – bread is not gf

Disclaimer: We do not guarantee, nor do these restaurants guarantee that any menu item will be 100% gluten-free. These restaurants & Business Graphics Group assume no liability for your use of this information. See full disclaimer on page 7.

Qdoba Mexican Grill

The following information about gluten-free menu items has been obtained either from the restaurant's website or through direct contact with guest services via email or phone.

List of Wheat-Free Menu Items (gluten is not listed on their allergen chart):

Rice and Beans:
Cilantro Lime Rice
Black Beans
Pinto Beans

Vegetables:
Fajita Vegetables
Grilled Vegetables
Romaine Lettuce

Taco Shells, Tortillas, Etc.:
Soft White Corn Tortilla

Proteins:
Pork
Chicken
Ground Sirloin
Seasoned Shredded Beef
Flat Iron Steak
Chorizo
Eggs

Salsas:
Pico de Gallo
Salsa Roja
Fiery Habanero
Salsa Verde
Roasted Chile Corn Salsa
Black Bean and Corn Salsa
Mango Salsa

Sauces:
Poblano Pesto
3-Cheese Queso
Ranchera
Guacamole
Lite Sour Cream
Cheese
Cilantro Lime Vinaigrette

Disclaimer: We do not guarantee, nor do these restaurants guarantee that any menu item will be 100% gluten-free. These restaurants & Business Graphics Group assume no liability for your use of this information. See full disclaimer on page 7.

Quiznos:

The following information about gluten-free menu items has been obtained either from the restaurant's website or through direct contact with guest services via email or phone.

Quiznos attempts to provide ingredient information regarding its products that is as complete as possible. The information contained in this document is based on standard product formulations. Variations may occur due to differences in suppliers, ingredient substitutions, recipe revisions, and/or product production at the restaurant. Some menu items may not be available at all restaurants; test products, test formulations or regional items may not be included. All items are prepared in common areas and may contain trace amounts of ingredients contained in other products.

Taco Salad with Chicken

Chopped salad no dressing

Buttermilk Ranch Dressing

Honey Mustard Dressing

Peppercorn Caesar Dressing

Raspberry Chipotle

Fat Free Balsamic

Fruit Parfait with Yogurt

Disclaimer: We do not guarantee, nor do these restaurants guarantee that any menu item will be 100% gluten-free. These restaurants & Business Graphics Group assume no liability for your use of this information. See full disclaimer on page 7.

Red Lobster

The menu items listed below do not contain wheat/gluten as an ingredient (includes all cooking sauces, condiments and fixed accompaniments).

Red Lobster has made every effort to ensure that the allergen information provided above is accurate. However, because of the handcrafted nature of our menu items, the variety of procedures used in our kitchens and our reliance on our suppliers, we can make no guarantees of its accuracy and disclaim liability for the use of this information. If you have any questions about this information, please ask to speak with a restaurant manager. This information is only valid June 1, 2010 through June 30, 2010. If you are dining after June 30, please contact us again for updated accurate information.

MENU ITEM LEGEND:
* Menu Item contains a Fried component (risk of cross contamination of all allergens)
**Menu item contains a Grilled component (risk of cross contamination of all allergens)
***Menu item contains a Fried and Grilled component (risk of cross contamination of all allergens)

Seaside Starters:
Lobster Nachos*

Regional Appetizers:
Buffalo Chicken Wings*

Dinner Entrees:
North Pacific King Crab Legs
Snow Crab Legs
Create Your Own Feast - Garlic Shrimp Scampi Create Your Own Feast - Steamed Snow Crab *Legs*
Create Your Own Feast - Wood-Grilled Fresh Fish**
Shrimp Your Way/Shrimp Lover's Monday & Tuesday
Scampi*

Lunch Entrees:
Farm-Raised Catfish - Blackened
Garlic Shrimp Scampi
Shrimp and Wood-Grilled Chicken - Garlic Shrimp *Scampi (with wild rice pilaf)***
Create Your Own Lunch - Garlic Shrimp Scampi

Add-On/Accompaniments:
Add Petite Shrimp to Your Salad
Baked Potato
Coleslaw
French Fries*
Freshly Cooked Potato Chips* (where available)
Home-Style Mashed Potatoes
Maine Lobster Tail Add-On
Roasted North Pacific King Crab Legs Add-On
Snow Crab Legs Add-On

Dressings/Sauces:
100% Pure Melted Butter
Add Butter to Baked Potato
Add Sour Cream to Baked Potato
Balsamic Vinaigrette
Blue Cheese Dressing
Caesar Dressing
French Dressing
Honey Mustard Dressing
Ketchup
Pico de Gallo
Ranch Dressing
Red Wine Vinaigrette
Tartar Sauce
Thousand Island Dressing

Disclaimer: We do not guarantee, nor do these restaurants guarantee that any menu item will be 100% gluten-free. These restaurants & Business Graphics Group assume no liability for your use of this information. See full disclaimer on page 7.

Red Lobster Continued:

Regional Lunch Entrees:
Walleye – Blackened

Promotional Items:
American Seafood Celebration

Kid's Menu:
Grilled Chicken**
Snow Crab Legs

Desserts:
New York-Style Cheesecake with Strawberries Surf' s Up Sundae

---

Disclaimer: We do not guarantee, nor do these restaurants guarantee that any menu item will be 100% gluten-free. These restaurants & Business Graphics Group assume no liability for your use of this information. See full disclaimer on page 7.

Red Robin

Recommended Menu Items for Guests with WHEAT/GLUTEN Allergies

Salads: (Dressings not included – see list of acceptable salad dressings)
Apple Harvest Chicken Salad - *No dijon vinaigrette, no candied walnuts, no bleu cheese crumbles or other cheese*
Cobb Salad - *No bleu cheese crumbles, no black olives, no garlic bread*
Crispy Chicken Tender Salad- *No fried chicken tenders. Grilled chicken breast may be used as a substitute, no garlic bread*
Mighty Caesar Salad *No blackened chicken -grilled chicken and salmon are available options, no croutons*
Side Caesar Salad *No croutons, no garlic bread*
Dinner Salad *No tortilla strips*

Salad Dressings: Please verify with the Manager since dressing may vary from restaurant location and geographic area

Balsamic Vinaigrette, Creamy Caesar, Bleu Cheese, Honey-Mustard Poppyseed
Note: Bleu cheese crumbles may not be used as a cheese option for any burgers and/or entrées.

Burgers: *Refer to sides for available side options

Monster Burger *No bun. May make protein-style by substituting a lettuce wedge for a bun. No Red Robin Seasoning on beef patties*
RR Gourmet Cheeseburger *No bun, No Red Robin Seasoning on beef patty*
Guacamole Burger *No bun, No Red Robin Seasoning on beef patty*
RR Bacon Cheeseburger *No bun, No Red Robin Seasoning on beef patty*
Royal Red Robin Burger *No bun, No Red Robin Seasoning on beef patty*
California Chicken Burger *No bun*

Note: Bleu cheese crumbles may not be used as a cheese option for any burgers and/or entrées.

Ensenada Chicken Platter: *No Baja Ranch Dressing, No Ancho marinade on chicken breasts, No tortilla strips, No tortilla cups*

Available Sides (Adult & Kids)
- White rice
- Celery sticks
- Melon wedges
- Guacamole
- Mandarin oranges • Steamed veggies
- Salsa
- Dinner Salad (*no tortilla strips*)
- Plain Red Robin Steak Fries (*without Red Robin Seasoning or garlic-parmesan seasoning) do not contain any allergens; however, there is a risk they might be fried in a common fryer with the allergens you want to avoid – please ask!!!*)

Kid's Menu *Refer to sides for available side options: *Kids may also select from any items listed on the Wheat/Gluten menu as a whole (adult items) to custom design a wheat/gluten free meal for your child.*

Rad Burger :
With Beef Patty *No bun. May make protein-style by substituting a lettuce wedge for a bun. No Red Robin Seasoning on beef patty*
With Turkey Patty *No bun. May make protein-style by substituting a lettuce wedge for a bun*
Chick-on-a-Stick *No teriyaki sauce. No ranch dressing*

Disclaimer: We do not guarantee, nor do these restaurants guarantee that any menu item will be 100% gluten-free. These restaurants & Business Graphics Group assume no liability for your use of this information. See full disclaimer on page 7.

Red Robin Continued:

Other Favorite Burgers: *Refer to sides for available side options

Grilled Salmon Burger *No bun, No Country Dijon Sauce*
Grilled Turkey Burger *No bun, No chipotle mayo*
Lettuce Wrap Your Burger *No Red Robin Seasoning on beef patty*
Bruschetta Chicken Burger *No bun, No tomato-bruschetta salsa. Plain salsa may be used as a substitute*

THIS INFORMATION NOT VALID AFTER 6/1/10 (per website). Red Robin relied on our suppliers' statements of ingredients in deciding which products did not contain certain allergens. Suppliers may change the ingredients in their products or the way they prepare their products, so please check this list to make sure that the menu item you like still meets your dietary requirements. From time to time we may substitute products due to inventory shortages. We can't be sure that the substitute products will be free of the allergen you wish to avoid. As we cook, prepare, and serve your meal, the listed menu option may come in contact with the allergen you want to avoid. For example, we might cook the listed menu option on the same broiler as a menu item that contains the allergen you want to avoid. That's just the way our kitchen is set up. Red Robin cannot guarantee that any menu item will be prepared completely free of the allergen in question.

Disclaimer: We do not guarantee, nor do these restaurants guarantee that any menu item will be 100% gluten-free. These restaurants & Business Graphics Group assume no liability for your use of this information. See full disclaimer on page 7.

Rubio's Fresh Mexican Grill

The following information about gluten-free menu items has been obtained either from the restaurant's website or through direct contact with guest services via email or phone.

List of Wheat-Free Menu Items (gluten is not listed on their allergen chart):

Side Salad
Chipotle Ranch Dressing
Balsamic Dressing
Surfside citrus Dressing
Cheese Enchiladas
Carnitas Enchiladas
Pinto Beans
Black Beans
Guacamole

Rubio's does not guarantee any meal completely free of the listed allergens and food products. The following products are cooked in a shared fryer: Beer-Battered Fish, Tortilla Chips, Churros, Rice and Chicken Taquitos. At Rubio's, it is important that we serve safe food and ensure that our guests are aware that our food may contain some of these common allergens.

Disclaimer: We do not guarantee, nor do these restaurants guarantee that any menu item will be 100% gluten-free. These restaurants & Business Graphics Group assume no liability for your use of this information. See full disclaimer on page 7.

Ruby Tuesday

Endless Fresh Garden Bar

Gluten/Wheat Free Toppings:
Green peas, shredded cheddar cheese, shredded Parmesan cheese, diced ham, bacon bits, diced eggs, edamame, garbanzo beans, cottage cheese, dried cranberries, diced red peppers, feta cheese crumbles, beets, sliced black olives

Gluten/Wheat Free Dressings:
French, Italian, Balsamic Vinaigrette, Honey Mustard

Gluten/Wheat Free Garden Bar Salads:
Cucumber Salad
Asian Salmon Spinach Salad *(no wonton strips, no sesame-peanut dressing)*
Avocado Shrimp Salad *(no wonton strips, no avocado ranch dressing)*
Southwestern Beef Salad *(no tortilla chips, no southwestern ranch dressing)*

Handcrafted Burgers:
(no bun, no french fries)
Ruby's Classic Burger
Classic Cheeseburger
Bacon Cheeseburger
Brewmaster Burger *(no Boston barbecue sauce)*
Boston Blue Burger *(no onion straws, no Boston barbecue sauce)*
Smokehouse Burger *(no onion straws, no barbecue sauce)*
Alpine Swiss Burger
Three Cheese Burger
Bison Bacon Cheeseburger

Premium Sandwiches:
The Ultimate Chicken *(no bun, no french fries)*

Handcrafted Steaks: *(no onion straws)*
Petite Sirloin *(7 oz.)*
Rib Eye *(12 oz.)*
Cowboy Sirloin *(no Boston barbecue sauce)*
Top Sirloin *(9 oz.)*
Peppercorn Mushroom Sirloin *(no Parmesan cream sauce)*
Steak & Lobster Tail

Fork-Tender Ribs:
Memphis Dry Rub Ribs *(half rack/full-rack)*

Specialties:
Barbecue Grilled Chicken *(no barbecue sauce, no succotash)*
Chicken Bella *(no Parmesan cream sauce)*
Chicken Fresco *(no lemon-butter sauce)*

Premium Seafood:
Steak* & Lobster Tail
Asian Glazed Salmon *(no sesame-peanut sauce, no brown-rice pilaf)*
New Orleans Seafood *(no Parmesan cream sauce, no brown-rice pilaf)*

Kid's Menu:
Beef Mini Burgers *(no bun, no french fries)*
Chop Steak
Grilled Chicken

Brunch: *(no biscuits, no cookies)*
Berry Good Yogurt Parfait *(no granola)*
Steak* & Eggs *(no crêpe)*
Spinach & Mushroom Omelet *(no seasoned potatoes)*
Western Omelet *(no seasoned potatoes)*
Mini Benedicts – Steak *(no bun, no seasoned potatoes)*

Kid's Brunch: *(no biscuits, no cookies, no seasoned potatoes)*
Eggscellent Combo

Disclaimer: We do not guarantee, nor do these restaurants guarantee that any menu item will be 100% gluten-free. These restaurants & Business Graphics Group assume no liability for your use of this information. See full disclaimer on page 7.

Ruby Tuesday Continued:

Prime Burgers: *(no bun, no french fries)*
Triple Prime Burger
Triple Prime Cheddar Burger
Triple Prime Bacon Cheddar Burger
Triple Prime Havarti Burger

Signature Sides:
Sautéed Baby Portabella Mushrooms
Sugar Snap Peas
Fresh Steamed Broccoli
White Cheddar Mashed Potatoes
Baked Potato

Desserts:
Berry Good Yogurt Parfait *(no granola)*

NOTE: *Ruby Tuesday strives to ensure that every guest has a great dining experience, and that includes those with special dietary needs and medical requirements. For this reason, we have prepared these menu options based on information obtained from our food suppliers. Every effort Is made to keep this information current and accurate. However, ingredient changes may occur due to substitutions, preparation variation, and regional availability of products. We encourage you to use these menu options as a tool to help you make your dining choices and not to the exclusion of professional medical advice tailored to your specific needs. We will update these online menus as our menu selections, ingredients, and/or preparation techniques change. Please visit our website often for the most current allergen/sensitivity information available. Limited time offers and weekend specials have not been included in these menu options .Current as of 06/01/2010 go to rubytuesday.com to make sure this is the latest issuance.*

Disclaimer: We do not guarantee, nor do these restaurants guarantee that any menu item will be 100% gluten-free. These restaurants & Business Graphics Group assume no liability for your use of this information. See full disclaimer on page 7.

Salad Creations

The following information about gluten-free menu items has been obtained either from the restaurant's website or through direct contact with guest services via email or phone.

This allergen review, conducted by HEALTHY DINING, is based upon product and recipe information supplied by Salad Creations. This review does not account for cross-contamination that may occur (1) during preparation of the menu item or (2) as a result of substituting alternative products to those listed above.

All menu item salads contain gluten. Here is a list of individual ingredients that are gluten free

- Alfalfa Sprouts
- Artichoke Hearts
- Beets
- Black Beans
- Black Olives
- Carrots
- Celery
- Cheddar Cheese
- Corn
- Cucumbers
- Dressing: Low Fat Light Honey Dijon
- Dressing: House Balsamic Vinaigrette
- Dressing: Honey Dijon
- Dressing: Lime Chipotle Vinaigrette
- Dressing: Raspberry Vinaigrette
- Dried Cranberries
- Feta Cheese
- Frozen Peas
- Garbanzo Beans (Chick Peas)
- Gorgonzola Crumbles
- Green Bell Pepper
- Green Onions
- Ham
- Hardboiled egg
- Hearts of Palm
- Iceberg Salad Mix
- Jalapeno Slices
- Kidney Beans
- Mandarin Oranges
- Mushrooms
- Parmesean Cheese
- Pepperoncini Peppers
- Raisins
- Raspberries
- Red Onions
- Romaine Lettuce
- Shrimp
- Spinach
- Spring Mix
- Swiss Cheese
- Tomatoes

Disclaimer: We do not guarantee, nor do these restaurants guarantee that any menu item will be 100% gluten-free. These restaurants & Business Graphics Group assume no liability for your use of this information. See full disclaimer on page 7.

Shane's Rib Shack

The following information about gluten-free menu items has been obtained either from the restaurant's website or through direct contact with guest services via email or phone.

At Shane's a top priority is always the health and safety of our guests. As part of our commitment to you, our gluten free menu is based on product information provided by Shane's approved food manufactures. Every effort is made to keep this information current. However, it is possible that ingredient changes and substitutions may occur due to the differences in regional suppliers, recipe revisions, preparation techniques, and/or the season of the year. We also have been unable to investigate sources of cross-contamination. Certain menu items may vary from restaurant to restaurant and may not be available at all locations. Therefore, we cannot be held responsible for individual reactions to any products. We highly recommend that our guests with food allergies or special dietary needs consult with a restaurant manager prior to placing an order to ensure the posted information is accurate and represents the menu items sold at that particular location. Limited time offers, test products, or regional items have not been included in the menus.
*Please see, http://www.fritolay.com/fl/flstore/cgi-bin/nutrition_faqs.htm, for Lay's comments about glutens.

Plates: (*Please let us know that you do not want bread when you order a plate*)
Pork
BBQ Chicken
Half Chicken
Whole Chicken
Half Rack Ribs
Full Rack Ribs
Beef Brisket
Grilled Chicken Tenders

BBQ Sauce:
Shane's Original BBQ Sauce

Sides:
Baked Beans
Cole Slaw
Collard Greens
Corn on the Cob
Green Beans
Side Salad
Chips *

Salads:
(*Please let us know you do not want onion crisps or garlic toast*)
The Shack (Pork or BBQ Chicken)
Grilled Chicken
Beef Brisket

Shane's logo spec dressing is gluten-free.

Disclaimer: We do not guarantee, nor do these restaurants guarantee that any menu item will be 100% gluten-free. These restaurants & Business Graphics Group assume no liability for your use of this information. See full disclaimer on page 7.

Sizzler

The following information about gluten-free menu items has been obtained either from the restaurant's website or through direct contact with guest services via email or phone.

Salad Bar Items:
Artichoke Hearts
Baby Corn
Bean Sprouts
Beets, Pickled
Bell Peppers, Green
Black Olives
Blue Cheese Crumbles
Broccoli Florets
Cantaloupe
Carrots
Cauliflower
Cheddar Cheese
Cherry Tomatoes
Cottage Cheese
Cucumbers
Eggs
Garbanzo Beans
Grapes
Green Beans
Green Onions
Honeydew Melon
Jicama
Kidney Beans
Mushrooms
Parmesan Cheese
Peas
Pineapple
Radishes
Raisins
Red Cabbage
Red Onions
Roasted Corn & Peppers
Romaine & Iceberg Lettuce Mix
Spinach
Spring Lettuce Mix
Strawberries
Sunflower Seeds
Turkey Ham
Watermelon
Zucchini

Salad Dressings:
Balsamic Vinaigrette
Signature Blue Cheese
Caesar
French
Italian
Low Fat Italian
Honey Mustard
Ranch Thousand Island

Prepared Salads:
Ambrosia Salad
Carrot Raisin Salad
Creamy Cole Slaw
Cucumber Tomato Salad
Green Salad
Potato Salad
Spinach Cranberry Salad
Srawberry Banana Salad
Three Bean Salad
Waldorf Salad

Sauces:
BBQ Sauce
Burger Sauce
Cocktail Sauce
Dill Tartar Sauce
Garlic Margarine
Honey Butter
Lemon Herb Sauce
Savory Butter

Soup:
Broccoli Cheese Soup
Chicken Tortilla Soup
Menudo

Disclaimer: We do not guarantee, nor do these restaurants guarantee that any menu item will be 100% gluten-free. These restaurants & Business Graphics Group assume no liability for your use of this information. See full disclaimer on page 7.

Sizzler Continued:

The nutritional and allergen information disseminated by Sizzler USA Restaurants, Inc. was prepared by Nutritional Information Services (www.nistn.com). The data contained herein was compiled from nutritional information and ingredient and allergen listings provided by our suppliers and distributors, and by an analysis generated using a software analysis program. NIS is the guarantor for the information provided. Sizzler USA Restaurants, Inc. and NIS assume no responsibility for errors in labeling or changes in the chemical or constituent composition of ingredients or prepared products used in Sizzler's recipes and menu items that are the direct or indirect result of the actions or inactions of the suppliers, distributors, and purveyors of said ingredients and products. The information within this guide is meant to provide a general estimate of the nutritional values associated with our menu items. The actual nutritional values may vary from the values listed due to variations in portion size(s), product preparation, and/or substitution of ingredients. The nutritional and allergen information provided is based upon the recipes being used at the time the guide was produced.

Recipes and menu items may be revised or changed from time to time, which affects the nutritional values. In addition, testing of new recipes for existing products may be conducted from time to time in certain markets. These new recipes may contain different/additional ingredients, including allergens, as compared to the original version. Some Sizzler locations may serve menu items which are not listed within this guide. Sizzler cannot guarantee that the nutritional information provided is completely accurate as it relates to the prepared menu items. If you have any questions or concerns about this nutritional and allergen information, or if you are sensitive to specific ingredients, please send us an email through the Contact Us page at www.sizzler.com. © 2010 Sizzler USA

Disclaimer: We do not guarantee, nor do these restaurants guarantee that any menu item will be 100% gluten-free. These restaurants & Business Graphics Group assume no liability for your use of this information. See full disclaimer on page 7.

Smokey Bones Bar and Fire Grill

The following information about gluten-free menu items has been obtained either from the restaurant's website or through direct contact with guest services via email or phone.

Guests with Gluten Sensitivities

Guests often contact us regarding what is safe for them to eat at Smokey Bones in regards to their Gluten Sensitivities (or Celiac Disease/Celiac Sprue). Gluten is a protein found in wheat, barley and rye. Smokey Bones has devised this list of menu items for our guests with gluten sensitivities. The items have been reviewed by an independent registered dietitian and determined generally to be suitable for consumption by the Gluten Intolerant, based upon the 2000 American Dietetic Association guidelines and menu samples provided by Smokey Bones. While Smokey Bones has made an effort to provide complete and current gluten content information, changes in recipes, and the handcrafted nature of our menu items mean that variations in the ingredient profile of a particular menu item may occur from time to time. Therefore, we make no guarantees regarding the gluten content of any of these items. Menu items should be ordered with recommended sides only with NO BREAD.

Fire starters:
Fire Stix
Smoked Wings

Salads and Soups:
Side Green Salad, crisp salad greens, with grape tomatoes, red onion, cucumbers (*NO CROUTONS*)
Side Caesar Salad(*NO CROUTONS*)
Charbroiled Chicken Caesar Salad (*NO CROUTONS*)
Cobb Salad
Country Potato Soup Cup and Bowl
Nutty Grilled Chicken Salad

Fire Grilled Steaks:
7oz Top Sirloin (*None Chipotle Marinated*)
10 oz Top Sirloin (*None Chipotle Marinated*)
12 oz NY Strip Steak
7 oz Filet Steak
All Toppings *Except Mushroom Sauce*

Chicken and Seafood:
BBQ ¼ Chicken
BBQ ½ Chicken
Fish and Chips
Bones Blackened Grouper
Grouper Grilled
Flamed Seared Salmon Teriyaki

Smoked BBQ:
Smoked St. Louis Style Ribs, All sizes with Original, Brown Sugar or Memphis Spice
Baby Back Ribs, All sizes with Original, Brown Sugar or Memphis Spice
Smoked Beef Brisket
Sliced Smoked Turkey breast

Sides:
Coleslaw
Broccoli
Apples
Mashed potatoes *WITHOUT gravy*
Loaded mashed potatoes
Baked potato
Loaded baked potato

Disclaimer: We do not guarantee, nor do these restaurants guarantee that any menu item will be 100% gluten-free. These restaurants & Business Graphics Group assume no liability for your use of this information. See full disclaimer on page 7.

Sonic

The following information about gluten-free menu items has been obtained either from the restaurant's website or through direct contact with guest services via email or phone.

*** Fried items are not always fried in designated stations. Fryer oil may come into contact with items containing milk, egg, fish, soy and wheat.
**** Blended / mixed drink items may come into contact with milk, egg, soy, wheat and peanuts.
Products containing allergens (e.g. milk, egg, fish, soy, peanuts, tree nuts and wheat, etc.) are used in this restaurant and may come in contact with your food or drink.

List of menu items without gluten

Grill Items:

- Hamburger Patty
- Hot Dog
- Steak
- Egg
- Bacon
- Breakfast Sausage

Fry Items:
*** French Fries (*see note about fried items, may be cross-contaminated*)
*** Tater tots (*see note about fried items, may be cross-contaminated*)

Cheese:

- Sliced American Cheese
- Shredded Cheddar Cheese
- Shredded Colby Jack Cheese

Other:

- Fritos
- Jalapenos
- Roasted corn and black bean
- Sliced Dill Pickles
- Green Chili Peppers
- Sliced
- Apple Slices

Salad Dressing/Condiments:

- Ranch Dressing
- Reduced Calorie Ranch
- Thousand Island Dressing
- Fat Free Italian
- Honey Mustard Dressing
- Relish sweet
- Ketchup
- Mustard
- Mayonnaise
- Honey Mustard Sauce
- Ranch dressing package
- Hickory BBQ Sauce
- Taco Sauce
- Tarter Sauce
- Maple Flavored Syrup
- Caramel Dipping Sauce
- mustard package
- Grape Jelly
- Strawberry Jam
- Marinara Sauce
- French Fry Sauce
- Sweet and sour sauce
- Picante Sauce

Disclaimer: We do not guarantee, nor do these restaurants guarantee that any menu item will be 100% gluten-free. These restaurants & Business Graphics Group assume no liability for your use of this information. See full disclaimer on page 7.

Sonic Continued:

Shakes, Drinks & Toppings:
(Blended / mixed drink items may come into contact with milk, egg, soy, wheat and peanuts.)

Soft Serve (Vanilla)	1% chocolate milk	1% Milk
Whipped Dessert Topping	Butterfinger	M & M
Reese's	Neutral Slush Base	Cherry Syrup
Diet Cherry Syrup	Grape Syrup	Blue Coconut Syrup
Bubble Gum Syrup	Orange Syrup	Cream pie syrup
Green Apple Syrup	Watermelon Syrup	Maraschino Cherries
Pineapple Topping	Strawberry Topping	Caramel topping
Butterscotch topping	Chocolate Syrup	Peanut butter
Nut Topping	Chocolate Fudge Topping	Hot Chocolate
Cocoa Mix		
Smoothie Powder	Coffee Creamer	Hazelnut
Raspberry Tea	Peach Tea	Blackberry Tea
Lemon Juice		

*** Fried items are not always fried in designated stations. Fryer oil may come into contact with items containing milk, egg, fish, soy and wheat. ***Products containing allergens (e.g. milk, egg, fish, soy, peanuts, tree nuts and wheat, etc.) are used in this restaurant and may come in contact with your food or drink.

Disclaimer: We do not guarantee, nor do these restaurants guarantee that any menu item will be 100% gluten-free. These restaurants & Business Graphics Group assume no liability for your use of this information. See full disclaimer on page 7.

Starbucks

The following information about gluten-free menu items has been obtained either from the restaurant's website or through direct contact with guest services via email or phone.

We do offer some packaged food items that meet gluten-free requirements including:

Kind Bars
Lucy's Cookies
Peeled Snacks
Two Mom's Raw Granola
Food Should Taste Good Chips

Starbucks is unable to guarantee a "gluten-free" environment in our retail locations due to the potential for cross contamination with gluten-containing products. The open environment and operating procedures of our store locations may present additional risk for gluten-sensitive customers aside from the gluten-containing ingredients themselves. "Gluten-free" is a claim with specific requirements defined by government agencies and industry standards. We are unable to make this claim on a product unless the item is specifically formulated and manufactured to meet the definition of the claim.

Please note that product assortment varies from location to location, and our packaged food offerings may change from season to season. If a packaged food item qualifies as gluten-free, it will be indicated on the label.

Disclaimer: We do not guarantee, nor do these restaurants guarantee that any menu item will be 100% gluten-free. These restaurants & Business Graphics Group assume no liability for your use of this information. See full disclaimer on page 7.

Subway

The following information about gluten-free menu items has been obtained either from the restaurant's website or through direct contact with guest services via email or phone.

Avoid the bread, bread is not gluten-free.

Salads: With lettuce, cucumbers, tomatoes, green peppers, red onions, olives and carrots
Chicken and Bacon Ranch (Includes Cheese)
Cold Cut Combo
Ham (Black Forest)
Italian BMT ®
Oven Roasted Chicken
Roast Beef
Tuna
Turkey Breast
Turkey Breast and Ham
Spicy Italian
Subway Club ®
Steak and Cheese
Veggie Delite ®

Meat, Poultry, Seafood and Eggs:
Bacon Strips
Oven Roasted Chicken
Chicken Strips – Plain
Cold Cut Combo meats
Egg (Regular) Omelet
Egg (White) Omelet
Ham (Black Forest)
Italian BMT ® meats
Roast Beef
Steak
Tuna
Turkey Breast

Cheese:
American Cheese
Cheddar Cheese
Monterey Cheddar Cheese, shredded
Parmesan Cheese
Pepperjack Cheese
Provolone Cheese
Swiss Cheese

Condiments and Dressings:
Chipotle Southwest Sauce
Honey Mustard Sauce
Light Mayonnaise/Regular Mayonnaise
Mustard (Yellow and Deli Brown)
Ranch Dressing
Red Wine Vinaigrette
Sweet Onion Sauce
Oil
Vinegar

Vegetables:
Banana Peppers
Jalapenos
Olives
Pickles
Vegetables (fresh)

Disclaimer: We do not guarantee, nor do these restaurants guarantee that any menu item will be 100% gluten-free. These restaurants & Business Graphics Group assume no liability for your use of this information. See full disclaimer on page 7.

Taco Bell

The following information about gluten-free menu items has been obtained either from the restaurant's website or through direct contact with guest services via email or phone.

Beverages:
Cherry Limeade Sparkler
Classic Limeade Sparkler
Classic Margarita Frutista Freeze

Sides:
Mexican Rice
Pintos & Cheese

Sauces:
Border Sauce – Fire
Border Sauce – Hot
Border Sauce – Mild
Creamy Jalapeno Sauce
Fiesta Salsa
Guacamole
Pepper Jack Sauce
Pizza Sauce
Red Sauce
Reduced Fat Sour Cream
Salsa
Spicy Avocado Ranch Dressing

Suggestions for Wheat and Gluten Sensitive Individuals:
Tostada
Fiesta Taco Salad (*order Chicken instead of Beef; order without the shell and without the Red Strips*)
Express Taco Salad (*order Chicken instead of Beef*)

The allergen information displayed on this page is based on standard product formulations and is current as of June 8, 2008 per website visit 5/2010. Variations may occur due to differences in suppliers, ingredient substitutions, recipe revisions, and/or product production at the restaurant.
Customers with allergy-related questions can contact the Food Allergy and Anaphylaxis Network (FAAN) on the web at foodallergy.org or by telephone at (800) 929-4040.

We fry our nacho chips and red strips in our restaurants. Our nacho chips and red strips DO NOT contain wheat, but the red strips and nacho chips are fried in the same fryer in which wheat-containing items are prepared. Some items on the "Gluten Containing" list contain oats (specifically Beef, Chili, and Taco Shell). Some individuals with Celiac Sprue may be able to consume oats.

Our new Frutista Freeze Strawberry and Mango beverages do not contain gluten. However, the strawberry topping used on the beverage is prepared in common equipment that may be in contact with gluten containing products.

If you have any further questions, or we can be of additional assistance, please contact us at the address or phone number listed below.
Taco Bell Corp., 17901 Von Karman, Mail Drop CS06, Irvine, CA 92614
Attn.: Consumer Inquiries
1-800-TACOBELL
www.tacobell.com

Disclaimer: We do not guarantee, nor do these restaurants guarantee that any menu item will be 100% gluten-free. These restaurants & Business Graphics Group assume no liability for your use of this information. See full disclaimer on page 7.

Ted's Montana Grill

For Those Needing a Gluten-Free Diet: *The kitchen at Ted's Montana Grill is not gluten-free but every attempt is made to meet your gluten-free needs. The analysis is based on the information available at time of publication. The following menu items are prepared with gluten-free products or can be ordered with the suggested changes to be gluten-free. Always request to speak with the manager when ordering.*

Starters:
Grilled Shrimp (*order without bread*)

Salads: *Please order your salad without croutons, as these do contain gluten.*
Grilled Caesar Salad (chicken, beef, bison, salmon or shrimp)
Chopped Salad
House Salad
Vine-Ripened Tomato and Onion Salad
Grilled Salad (chicken, beef, bison, salmon or shrimp)
Wedge
Caesar Side Salad

Dressings: Caesar, Honey Mustard, Creamy Vinaigrette, Bleu Cheese and Thousand Island Dressings are gluten-free.

Burgers and Chicken Sandwiches: (*order without the bun*)
USDA Choice Beef, Great Range Brand BisonTM or All-Natural Chicken. Served with our fresh-cut French fries.

Naked	Philly	George's Cadillac
Green & Hot	Kitchen Sink	Spikebox
S.O.B.	C.O.B.	Swiss & Mushroom
Ultimate Skinny Dip	Bleu Creek	Skinny Dip
Cheese	Vermejo	
New Mexico	America's Cup	

Entrées: (*order without yeast roll*)
Please refer to the listing of gluten-free sides when ordering your entrée.
Cedar Plank Salmon
Bison or Beef Delmonico
Prime Rib (*order without au jus*)
Roast Turkey (*order without dressing and gravy*)
Bison or Beef Tenderloin Filet
Brick Chicken
Bison Kansas City Strip Steak
Beer Can Chicken (*order without chicken jus*)

Kids' Menu:
Please refer to the listing of gluten-free sides when ordering your entrée.
Bar None Sliders[SM] (*order without roll*)
Cedar Plank Salmon

Disclaimer: We do not guarantee, nor do these restaurants guarantee that any menu item will be 100% gluten-free. These restaurants & Business Graphics Group assume no liability for your use of this information. See full disclaimer on page 7.

Ted's Montana Grill Continued:

Sides:

Asparagus	Cottage Cheese	Mashed Potatoes
Broccoli	Cole Slaw	Baked Potato
Vine-Ripened Tomatoes	French Fries	Sweet Potato

Desserts:
Häagen-Dazs® Ice Cream
Root Beer or Coke Float
Shakes

Disclaimer: We do not guarantee, nor do these restaurants guarantee that any menu item will be 100% gluten-free. These restaurants & Business Graphics Group assume no liability for your use of this information. See full disclaimer on page 7.

Tony Roma's

The following information about gluten-free menu items has been obtained either from the restaurant's website or through direct contact with guest services via email or phone.

Ribs
Grilled Chicken
Steaks
Grilled Fish
Barbecue Sauce

It is important for our valued guest to know our fry oil is shared with gluten products and cross-contamination is an expectation and evident in any fried item such as chicken tenders, French fries, tortilla chips, etc.

Disclaimer: We do not guarantee, nor do these restaurants guarantee that any menu item will be 100% gluten-free. These restaurants & Business Graphics Group assume no liability for your use of this information. See full disclaimer on page 7.

Uno's Chicago Grill

The following information about gluten-free menu items has been obtained either from the restaurant's website or through direct contact with guest services via email or phone.

UNO Chicago Grill goes to tremendous strides to identify all forms of gluten and gluten derivatives in the foods we purchase or prepare in house... however, we cannot be responsible for individual reactions to any food products or guarantee that the food we serve is free from any allergen. UNO Chicago Grill is providing this information for educational purposes only. In no way should it be considered medical advice. UNO Chicago Grill disclaims all responsibility related to the use of this information. If you have any questions regarding whether eating particular foods may cause an allergic reaction for you, please speak with your physician.

Smoke, Sizzle & Splash:
Top Sirloin Steak
New York Strip Steak
Chop House Classic
Lemon Basil Salmon
Baby Back Ribs

Grilled Mahi-Mahi with Mango Salsa

Pizza: *(specify gluten-free)*
Gluten Free Cheese Pizza
Gluten Free Pepperoni Pizza
Gluten Free Veggie Pizza

Chicken:
Grilled Rosemary Chicken
Grilled Chicken with Mango Salsa
Grilled Chicken Breast

Great Greens:
House Salad
Classic Cobb Salad
Caesar Salad
Chicken Caesar Salad

Dressing choices: Balsamic Vinaigrette or Caesar

Burgers: *(no bun)*
The Uno Burger
Kid's Cheeseburger

Available Toppings: peppers, onion, mushrooms, bacon or cheddar

Sides:
Brown Rice with Ocean Spray®
Sweetened Dried Cranberries and Mango
Red Bliss Mashed Potato
Steamed Broccoli
Steamed or Roasted Seasonal Vegetables

Beer: Redbridge

Drinks:
Harney Artisan Organic Tea
Fresh Lemonade
Freshly-Brewed Lipton Iced Tea

Freezers:
Strawberry Smoothie
Chocolate Monkey
Tropical Fruit Freezer
Raspberry Lime Ricky
Wildberry Mango Smoothie

Desserts:
Ice Cream Sundae
(Vanilla ice cream w/ chocolate sauce)

For a more comprehensive listing of nutritionals and ingredient statements, please go back to Main Menu and select individual menu items. Please Note: Nutritionals and ingredient statements do not reflect substitutions and/or changes made to accommodate gluten free preerences.

Disclaimer: We do not guarantee, nor do these restaurants guarantee that any menu item will be 100% gluten-free. These restaurants & Business Graphics Group assume no liability for your use of this information. See full disclaimer on page 7.

Wendy's

U.S. Menu Items Without Gluten: *No Wheat, Barley, Oats, or Rye*
*Ingredient information is based on standard product formulations. Variations may occur due to differences in suppliers, ingredient substitutions, recipe revisions, product assembly at the restaurant level, and/or the season of the year. Certain menu items may not be available at all locations. Temporary products are not included. This information is effective as of **June, 2010.** Wendy's International, Inc., its franchisees and employees do not assume responsibility for a particular allergy or sensitivity to any food provided in our restaurants. We encourage anyone with food allergies, sensitivities, or special dietary needs to check our website at www.wendys.com on a regular basis to obtain the most comprehensive and up-to-date information. If you have specific questions about our menu, call or write: Wendy's International, Inc., Consumer Relations Department, One Dave Thomas Boulevard, Dublin, OH 43017-0256, 614-764-3100.*

Meats:
Hamburger Patty
Grilled Chicken Breast+

Condiments:
American Cheese
Applewood Smoked Bacon
Bacon Jr.
Buttery Best Spread+
Cheddar Cheese Sauce
Dill Pickles
Honey Mustard Sauce
Ketchup
Iceberg Lettuce Leaf
Mustard
Natural Swiss Cheese
Onion
Ranch Sauce
Reduced Fat Sour Cream+
Tomato
Tartar Sauce*

Salads:
Caesar Side Salad
(*without croutons*)
Side Salad
Baja Salad
Seasoned Tortilla Strips+
Southwest Taco Salad
Seasoned Tortilla Strips+
Reduced Fat Sour Cream+

Dressings:
Ancho Chipotle Ranch Dressing*
Avocado Ranch Dressing*
Classic Ranch Dressing*
Creamy Red Jalapeno Dressing*
Fat Free French Dressing*
Honey Dijon Dressing*
Italian Vinaigrette Dressing*
Lemon Garlic Caesar Dressing*
Light Classic Ranch Dressing*
Pomegranate Vinaigrette Dressing*
Supreme Caesar Dressing*
Thousand Island Dressing*

Baked Potatoes:
Plain
Sour Cream & Chives
Bacon & Cheese*
Broccoli & Cheese*
Chili & Cheese*

Side Items:
Chili
Hot Chili Seasoning Packet
Cheddar Cheese, shredded
Mandarin Orange Cup

Frosty™:
Chocolate Frosty
Vanilla Frosty
Coffee Toffee Twisted Frosty
M&M's® Twisted Frosty
Chocolate Fudge Frosty Shake
Frosty™ -cino
Strawberry Frosty Shake
Vanilla Bean Frosty Shake

Disclaimer: We do not guarantee, nor do these restaurants guarantee that any menu item will be 100% gluten-free. These restaurants & Business Graphics Group assume no liability for your use of this information. See full disclaimer on page 7.

Wendy's Continued:

Beverages:
Coffee
Iced Tea
Hot Tea
Sweet Tea*
Coca-Cola®
Diet Coke®
Sprite®
Barq's® Root Beer*
Coke Zero™*
Dr Pepper®
Fanta® Orange*
Hi-C® Flashin' Fruit Punch*
Minute Maid® Light Lemonade*
Pibb Xtra®*
Dasani® Water*
Nesquik® Low Fat Chocolate Milk
Nesquik Low Fat White Milk

French Fries may be cooked in the same oil as Boneless Chicken Wings, Crispy Chicken Patty, Crispy Chicken Nuggets, Spicy Chicken Nuggets (where available) & Fish Fillets (where available), which contain a wheat allergen.

Coca-Cola, Coke Zero, Dasani, Diet Coke, Fanta, Hi-C, Minute Maid, Pibb Xtra and Sprite are trademarks of The Coca-Cola Company. Barq's is a registered trademark of Barq's, Inc. M&M's is a registered trademark of Mars, Incorporated. Nesquik is a registered trademark of Société Des Produits Nestlé S.A., Vevey, Switzerland. Dr Pepper is a registered trademark of Dr Pepper/Seven Up, Inc.
*Certain menu items may vary from store to store and may not be available at all locations.
+Contains maltodextrin from a corn source.
This list may not be published or distributed in any manner without prior written consent of Wendy's International, Inc. © 2010 Oldemark LLC. The Wendy's name, design and logo, and Frosty are trademarks of Oldemark LLC and are licensed to Wendy's International, Inc.

Disclaimer: We do not guarantee, nor do these restaurants guarantee that any menu item will be 100% gluten-free. These restaurants & Business Graphics Group assume no liability for your use of this information. See full disclaimer on page 7.

Wingstop

The following information about gluten-free menu items has been obtained either from the restaurant's website or through direct contact with guest services via email or phone.

*All Wings * (except boneless wing strips – as these are breaded)*
All Sauces are gluten free
All Side Dishes are gluten free

* Even though our wings are not breaded, there is a possibility that our wings could be fried in shortening that had also fried our breaded wing strips. Therefore there is a possibility that our wings may contain some gluten from frying in the same shortening.

Disclaimer: We do not guarantee, nor do these restaurants guarantee that any menu item will be 100% gluten-free. These restaurants & Business Graphics Group assume no liability for your use of this information. See full disclaimer on page 7.

Disclaimer: We do not guarantee, nor do these restaurants guarantee that any menu item will be 100% gluten-free. These restaurants & Business Graphics Group assume no liability for your use of this information. See full disclaimer on page 7.

Made in the USA
Charleston, SC
15 September 2010